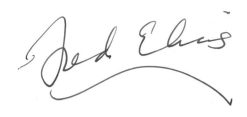

DIFFUSE PULMONARY DISEASE

A Radiologic Approach

IRWIN M. FREUNDLICH, M.D.

Professor of Radiology,
University of Arizona, Tucson, Arizona

1979

W. B. SAUNDERS COMPANY / Philadelphia / London / Toronto

W. B. Saunders Company: West Washington Square
Philadelphia, PA   19105

1 St. Anne's Road
Eastbourne, East Sussex BN21 3UN, England

1 Goldthorne Avenue
Toronto, Ontario M8X 5T9, Canada

Library of Congress Cataloging in Publication Data

Freundlich, Irwin M

Diffuse pulmonary disease.

1. Lungs — Diseases — Diagnosis.   2. Lungs — Radiography.
   I. Title.

RC734.R3F65   616.2'4'0757   77–27745

ISBN 0–7216–3866–X

Diffusion Pulmonary Disease   ISBN   0-7216-3866-X

Last digit is the print number: 9   8   7   6   5   4   3   2   1

This book is dedicated to those radiologists and other physicians who have studied, investigated, and written about diseases of the chest.

Preface

This book is meant to be a sequel to Felson's *Principles of Chest Roentgenology, A Programed Text,* although the format is quite different. It is not quasi-programmed or even semiprogrammed but is arranged so that the reader may first see the method and how it is applied and then test himself or herself on a series of cases of increasing difficulty. Although the initial intent included programming, it was finally rejected, as I believe this method tends to lead the observer. Radiographs do not come across the stack with multiple-choice questions attached. To be sure, the difficulty of programming a text played a role in this decision as well.

The case material involves diffuse pulmonary disease in children and adults, but not the pulmonary problems of the neonate, which constitute an entirely different subject. Because of the nature of diffuse pulmonary disease, lateral examinations of the chest are less helpful than with other pulmonary problems, and relatively few are included in this book. However, the lateral projection should not be omitted as part of the routine radiographic examination of the chest.

It is always difficult to acknowledge those individuals to whom the author of a textbook is indebted, because so many must be left out. However, the importance of the environment in which any work is done cannot be over-estimated. The very positive influence of the Department of Radiology at the University of Arizona is largely due to its chairman, Dr. Paul Capp. It has been my privilege to have been part of this department since its first day, and it is a place which is conducive to good radiology in all its aspects.

I should also like to thank Dr. Bob Campbell of Philadelphia, whose invitation to give a refresher course at the R.S.N.A. meeting finally led to the organization of this material, and Dr. Mike Pitt of our department, whose critical review of the text was most helpful. Many radiology residents have contributed over the years to this approach to diffuse pulmonary disease, but I would like to thank particularly Drs. Anna Nussbaum, Frederick Park, and Randall Stickney for their help in reviewing the material from the resident's point of view. The quality of the photographs is due directly to the diligence and attention to detail of Mark Henry and Cliff Pollack of our Audiovisual Division. The hours spent in making sure the photographs were of the highest quality are much appreciated. Last but certainly not least is Ms. Janet Quinones, able assistant, tireless typist, and guardian of the gate, whose long hours of dedication to the task were surpassed only by her good humor in carrying it out.

IRWIN M. FREUNDLICH, M.D.

University of Arizona
May, 1978

v

Contents

Introduction

All textbooks, whether in radiology or another discipline, are written with a specific purpose in mind. One such purpose would be to compile a reference book containing a description of all the diseases afflicting a certain organ system; another might be to write a monograph expounding on a single disease entity, and a third would be to teach a method of carrying out and interpreting certain procedures. In the *practice* of radiology, however, one begins with the discovery of a problem, and after the discovery, proceeds with the differential diagnosis. A realistic and practical method of instruction, therefore, is to teach an *approach* to the problem. This book is such an attempt; the problem is diffuse pulmonary disease.

When a resident or student asks how to approach diffuse pulmonary disease, the physician often answers, "Carefully" or "As seldom as possible" with a nervous chuckle. All too often radiographic reports of diffuse pulmonary disease are merely descriptive and make no attempt to arrive at a differential diagnosis. In defense of such descriptions it must be acknowledged that the lung has a limited capacity to respond to injury, and therefore many diseases present similar patterns. There are, however, too many reports of "hazy densities at the bases" or "increased markings" without any attempt at a differential diagnosis. Reports limited to description are less than adequate.

Radiologists are often helpless without some clinical information, and this is nowhere more true than when they are at-tempting a diagnosis of diffuse pulmonary disease. The radiologist must request of the clinicians with whom he works the basic clinical data in each case. In approaching diffuse pulmonary disease one needs to marshall all available help, clinical data as well as the radiologic gamut, to sally forth and meet the enemy, to accept the "challenge of the radiograph."

Pulmonary parenchymal disease can be divided generally into local and diffuse processes. Usually this differentiation is a simple one, but occasionally diseases that under ordinary circumstances would be manifested only in a limited area of the lung, become widespread. For example, bacterial pneumonia and reinfection tuberculosis are local disease processes, but at times they may involve the entirety of both lungs. This book deals primarily with those diseases that are most often diffuse in nature, although it certainly is true that there is a gray zone between diseases ordinarily considered to be local and those generally thought to be diffuse.

It has never done me much good to have a choice of 98 causes of diffuse pulmonary disease without some way to divide and conquer. Therefore, the approach presented in this book is essentially a process of elimination, one that uses an analysis of the roentgen findings and clinical information. Common diseases are stressed, particularly those that present acute life-threatening situations.

The approach is divided into five general sections, and, although there is some overlap, each section will be considered separately. In each of the five sections the approach is presented by a question or a statement, as follows:

Section A. Is the patient *immunosuppressed*, does he have a known neoplasm, or is he on steroid therapy?

Section B. Is the disease *multinodular?*

Section C. Is the disease predominantly an *airspace* filling process?

Section D. Is pulmonary *hyperaeration* and/or pulmonary *arterial hypertension* the dominant feature?

Section E. The disease is *predominantly interstitial* but not grossly nodular. It may be granular, reticular, mottled, or linear, and any hyperaeration present is secondary.

Within each section a stepwise series of decisions synthesizing the diagnostic possibilities, the radiographic appearance, and the clinical data will be made. Each section is summarized diagrammatically, which many may find a useful way of retaining the information. Thereafter, in each section a series of cases will be presented; these can be used by the reader as unknowns to test the method and to test himself or herself in the evaulation of diffuse pulmonary disease. A discussion of each case will be found following the case presentation.

Is the patient immunosuppressed?

Does he have a known neoplasm?

Is he on steroid therapy?

Section A

If the answer to any of the three questions listed above is yes, we will work within the framework of Section A. While it is possible that the patient may have developed new pulmonary disease incidental to the suppression of his immune mechanisms, this is hardly likely and may be safely discounted as a possibility. New pulmonary disease in this type of patient invariably falls into one of the following categories:

    1. the neoplasm itself
    2. a reaction to drug therapy
    3. an opportunistic infection

Also to be considered are
    4. transfusion reaction
    5. radiation reaction

Decision 1. Is the new pulmonary disease caused by the neoplasm itself? (Many leukemic patients will fall into this category. Although leukemic pulmonary infiltrations noted radiographically are exceedingly rare, pulmonary hemorrhage secondary to platelet depletion and thrombocytopenia must be considered.) Primary pulmonary neoplasm, except for some cases of alveolar cell carcinoma, is almost always a local process, but the various manifestations of metastatic disease must be considered. These include the following:

a. *Hematogenous spread of carcinoma,* which usually produces multiple nodules but may also give rise to a lymphangitic component superimposed on the nodules.

b. *Lymphangitic distribution of carcinoma* emanating from one or both hila or the mediastinum. The lymphatics are dammed up as a result of hilar lymph node replacement but may actually contain neoplasm. Most of these neoplasms will be metastases from a primary carcinoma of the breast.

c. *Lymphangitic extension through the diaphragm* arising from, for example, carcinoma in the tail of the pancreas or the fundus of the stomach.

d. Diffuse pulmonary lymphoma on initial presentation is unusual and almost invariably is associated with lymphadenopathy. However, in the later stages of the disease, particularly following mediastinal radiation therapy, pulmonary lymphoma may be widespread in the absence of obvious hilar and mediastinal lymphadenopathy.

Decision 2. Is the patient's drug therapy directly responsible for the new pulmonary disease? As far as a reaction to chemotherapy is concerned, any patient may react in an idiosyncratic fashion to any drug. However, drugs that are well known causes of pulmonary reactions include:

    a. methotrexate
    b. busulfan
    c. phenytoin (Dilantin)
    d. nitrofurantoin
    e. bleomycin

Drugs such as Adriamycin and daunomycin must be added, but these are predominantly cardiotoxic drugs, and patients may present with the signs, symptoms, and roentgenographic picture of congestive heart failure.

Decision 3. The phrase "opportunistic infection" has been widely used to describe infection in the compromised host. The infecting organism, however, is often a pathogen but may indeed be a true opportunist. Infections in the compromised host fall into one of the following categories:

    a. bacterial
    b. viral
    c. fungal
    d. parasitic (*Pneumocystis carinii*)
    e. tuberculous

A bacterial infection that arises in an immunosuppressed host often begins as a local process, and the diagnosis may be established before diffuse disease ensues. We will not consider single or multiple areas of local infection in this text. One must bear in mind, however, that the picture of infection one is accustomed to see in the patient whose normal host defenses are intact may not be present in the immunosuppressed patient. This is particularly true in patients in whom the white cells are depleted and in whom a diffuse bacterial pneumonia may be the initial radiologic presentation.

Decision 4. This decision involves the possibility of an transfusion reaction, which is usually abrupt and occurs within an hour or 2 of the transfusion. Diagnosis must be made primarily on the history of a recent transfusion. The change in the patient's status as well as the change in the radiographic appearance is usually fairly dramatic. In the patient with a clear chest prior to transfusion, particularly a white cell transfusion, a reaction to blood products must be differentiated from pneumonia, which may not be seen in leukocyte-depleted patients until after transfusion.

Decision 5. A reaction to radiation may present a diagnostic problem, but often the shape of the portal previously employed can be seen on the radiograph, which simplifies the problem.

The radiographic appearance of the new pulmonary disease can now be evaluated based on the five categories just enumerated. In its appearance the disease will be nodular, an alveolar filling process, or linear. If the disease is nodular in the compromised host, then clearly one must consider either

    a. metastases or
    b. diffuse granulomatous infiltration.

As will be demonstrated, in metastatic carcinoma the nodules vary considerably in size and are well marginated, while diffuse granulomatous nodules are similar in size, and the margins of each are quite irregular. Diseases that present with multiple small granulomata in the compromised host are fungal infections and tuberculosis. Multiple large masses may also be seen with infections with specific organisms, such as *Nocardia,* and also, but rarely, with any of the fungi.

If the disease is an alveolar filling process, one must consider

    a. a drug reaction with cardiac failure
    b. a bacterial or fungal infection
    c. a transfusion reaction
    d. pulmonary hemorrhage

Drug reactions are widespread, or central and symmetric, while bacterial pneumonias tend to be peripheral in distribution. A central and symmetric alveolar filling disease may also be due to the failure of another organ system, cardiac or renal, or to a systemic response to an insult such as chemotherapy.

If the new disease is linear in its appearance (predominantly interstitial), then one should think of

    a. superimposed congestive heart failure (interstitial pulmonary edema)
    b. an early drug reaction
    c. lymphangitic spread of carcinoma
    d. a diffuse viral infection
    e. *Pneumocystis carinii* infection

Once again, if the process is central and symmetric, the early manifestations of pulmonary edema, whether secondary to a drug reaction, cardiac failure, or overhydration, must be considered.

In summary, the clinical data must be synthesized with the radiographic appearance of the disease and the best diagnostic possibilities derived from the decision-making process just described.

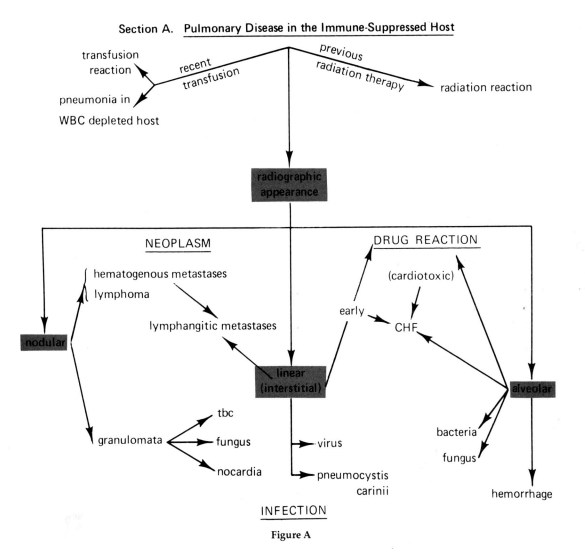

Section A. Pulmonary Disease in the Immune-Suppressed Host

Figure A

CASE A–1

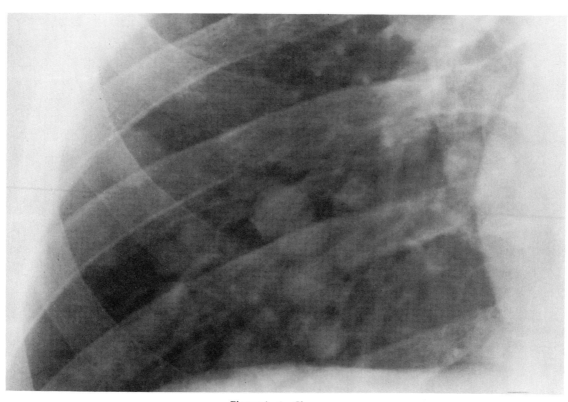

Figure A–1 Close-up

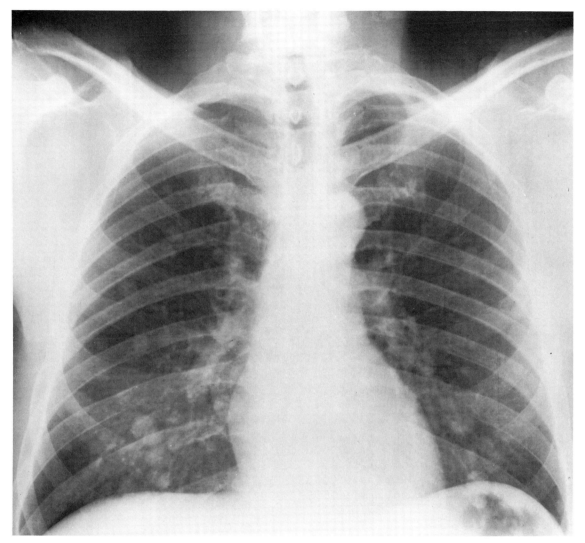

Figure A-1

Case A-1. This patient was a 51 year old black male who presented without respiratory symptomatology 8 months following surgery for a soft tissue angiosarcoma. The patient was not taking medication, and the chest radiographs were made as part of a routine examination.

DISCUSSION, CASE A–1

The patient has obvious multiple hematogenous metastases. However, the question of interest is, why is the case obvious? We recognize the lesions as metastatic because they are *multiple* and relatively *well circumscribed* and show a considerable *variation in size*. While most cases are obvious, at times multiple pulmonary metastases are quite small and superficially resemble diffuse granulomatous infection. Close observation in almost every case of metastases, however, reveals the variation in size and the relatively sharp outlines.

CASE A–2 _____

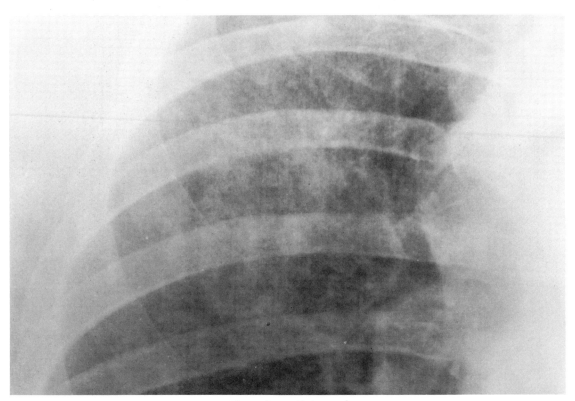

Figure A–2 Close-up

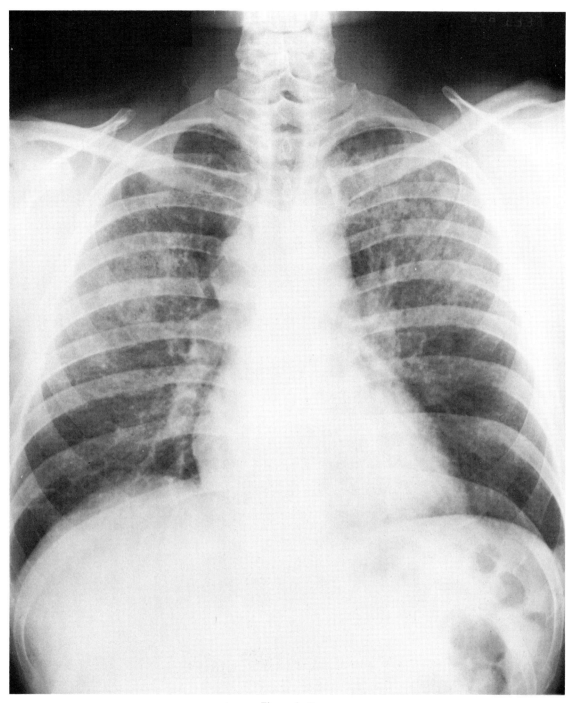

Figure A–2

Case A–2. This patient was a 41 year old white male who presented with 10 days of increasing dyspnea, cough, and fatigue. He had a known carcinoma of the nasopharynx with cerebral as well as mediastinal metastases. He was on methotrexate therapy as well as phenytoin (Dilantin) for seizure activity. Since neither radiation therapy nor a blood transfusion plays a role in this case, one must decide whether the new chest disease is caused by

1. the patient's known neoplasm
2. a drug reaction
3. opportunistic infection

DISCUSSION, CASE A–2

Did you note that the disease is bilateral, central, and relatively symmetric? What then is your choice for the best diagnostic possibility?

Pulmonary reaction to methotrexate or Dilantin, or both, is the best diagnosis. While these initial cases are relatively straightforward, application of the same principles will allow you to make the diagnosis more often than you would have thought possible. In this case the bilateral central and symmetric appearance strongly suggests a drug reaction rather than pulmonary infection or spread of the patient's neoplasm. The alveolar quality of the parenchymal infiltrations and the symmetric appearance rules against metastatic neoplasm, but some opportunistic infections cannot be entirely excluded, particularly *Pneumocystis carinii* infection. The patient was not treated except for elimination of the two drugs he was taking, and the new parenchymal disease cleared entirely within 10 days. The rapid clearing suggests that the reaction was probably due to Dilantin rather than to methotrexate.

CASE A–3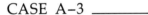

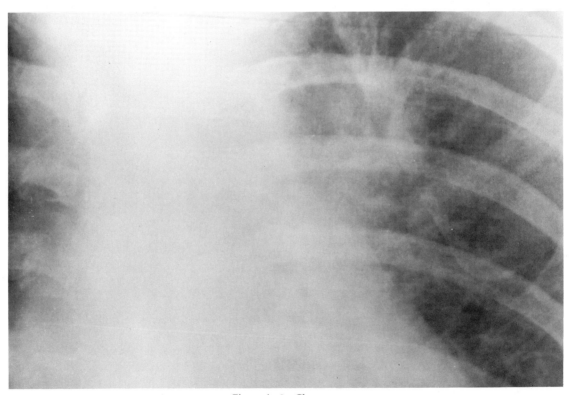

Figure A–3 Close-up

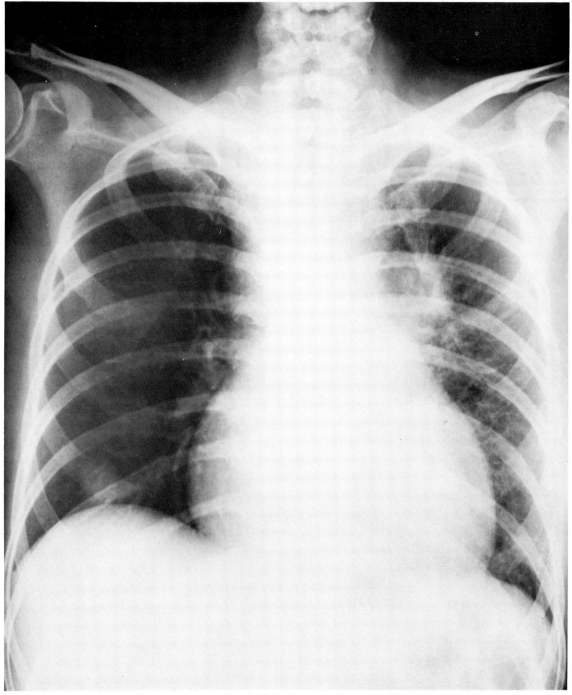

Figure A–3

Case A–3. This patient was a 46 year old white female who presented with dyspnea, headache, nausea, and vomiting. She had had a right mastectomy for carcinoma of the breast 2½ years previously, followed by radiation therapy to the right side. The patient was begun on methotrexate chemotherapy a few days prior to this radiograph. Is the new chest disease caused by

1. the known neoplasm
2. a drug reaction
3. opportunistic infection
4. radiation reaction

DISCUSSION, CASE A–3

After noting that there has been a mastectomy, one must initially ascertain whether the patient has received postoperative radiation therapy. Although it would be entirely unexpected to have a radiation reaction on the contralateral side and not the ipsilateral side, communication with the therapist, and if necessary, inspection of the portal film will enable you to determine whether the lung was treated. The asymmetry of the process also essentially rules out a drug reaction, which is expected to be either central and symmetric, or diffuse, but in either case bilateral.

The differential diagnosis in this case lies between an opportunistic pneumonitis and lymphangitic spread of the patient's known neoplasm. Which would you choose? If you chose lymphangitic spread of the patient's breast carcinoma, you are correct. Pneumonitis would have been more pronounced in the peripheral portion of the lung than in the central portion. Lymphangitic spread from a breast carcinoma in this fashion is relatively common but would be unusual for other types of neoplasm. There is probably direct lymphatic extension of carcinoma from the internal mammary lymphatics to the hilar lymph nodes on each side. Further observation in this case reveals probable mediastinal and hilar lymphadenopathy. Occasionally metastases from other primary tumors — for example, renal or testicular carcinoma — will involve mediastinal or hilar lymph nodes, or both, before the pulmonary parenchyma is involved. In these cases one may also see distended pulmonary lymphatics secondary to obstruction.

CASE A–4

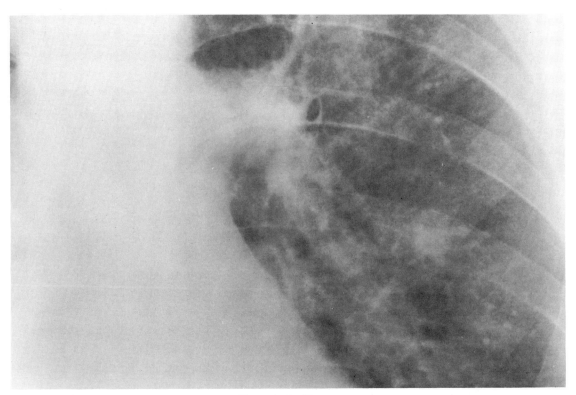

Figure A–4 Close-up

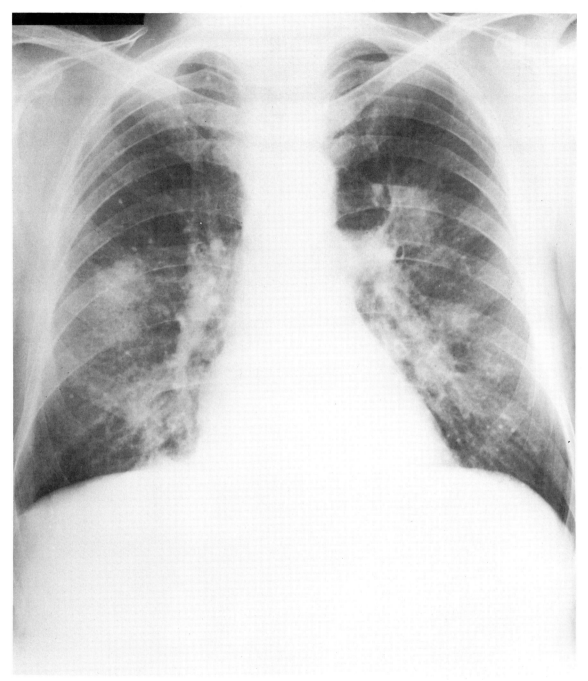

Figure A-4

Case A-4. This patient was a 47 year old white male who presented for a routine examination. He was known to have chronic myelogenous leukemia and was taking moderate doses of steroids. He complained only of a mild cough, occasionally productive of sputum. Is his new chest disease caused by

1. the known neoplasm
2. a drug reaction
3. opportunistic infection

DISCUSSION, CASE A–4

An opportunistic infection, in this case *Nocardial* infection, is the best possibility. Although microscopic leukemic infiltrations may be seen at autopsy, these are rarely visible macroscopically and would never present as multiple parenchymal masses. The multiple masses, therefore, are compatible only with opportunistic infection. The size of the masses as well as their indistinct borders suggests *Nocardial* infection, which often presents in this fashion and frequently cavitates. Opportunistic fungal infection would be the only other diagnosis worthy of consideration.

CASE A–5 _____

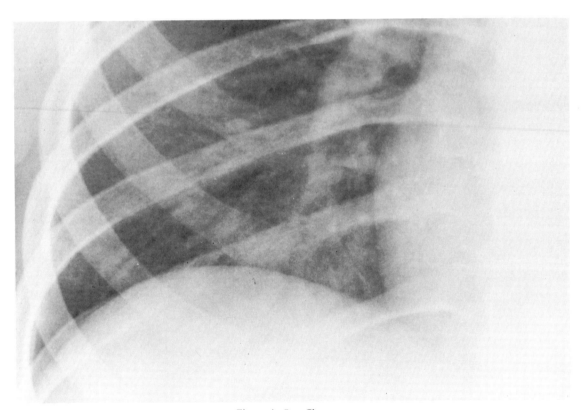

Figure A–5a Close-up

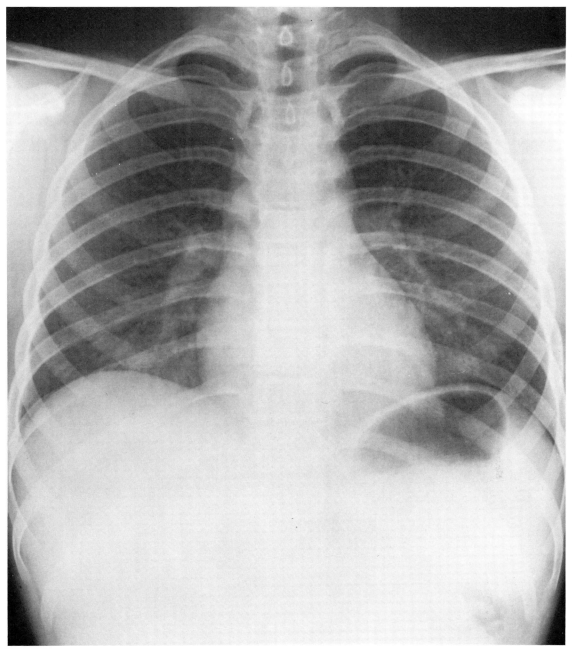

Figure A–5a

Case A–5a. This patient was a 15 year old white male who presented after 2 months of progressive dyspnea and a minimal cough. He had been under therapy for acute myelogenous leukemia for the past 2 years. The therapy included methotrexate, Cytoxan, vincristine, and prednisone, and he was at the time of admission in clinical remission. A radiograph made 1 week later is on the next page (Fig. A–5b).

CASE A–5 *CONTINUED*

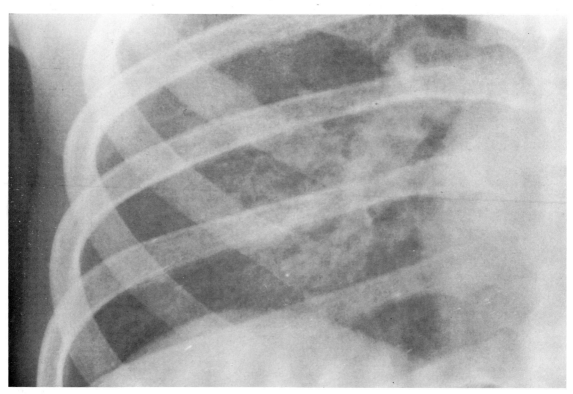

Figure A–5b   Close-up

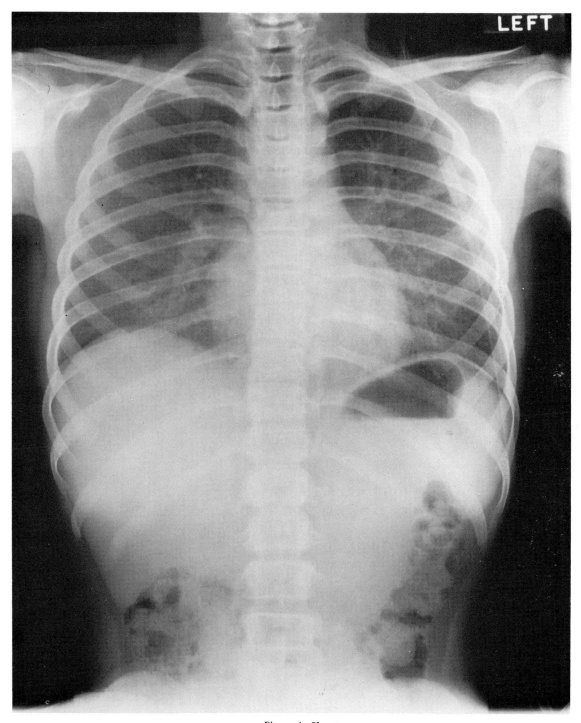

Figure A–5b

Case A–5b.   This radiograph is of the same patient demonstrated in Figure A–5a. All medications were stopped, but the patient continued to demonstrate increasing dyspnea and fatigue and was admitted to the hospital. There had been no recent blood transfusions. Is the patient's new chest disease caused by

1. the known neoplasm
2. a drug reaction
3. opportunistic infection

DISCUSSION, CASE A–5

If you made the diagnosis from the radiograph presented in Figure A–5a, you are doing very well indeed. Of course, the essential question about the first radiograph is whether it was a normal or an abnormal examination. However, 1 week later the diffuse fine interstitial process with partial obliteration of the vascular markings is much more apparent. Hypoaeration is also present. Biopsy revealed *Pneumocystis carinii* pneumonia, but therapy could not be instituted in time to save the patient from this opportunistic infection. The possibility of a drug reaction must be considered in this case, but whenever *Pneumocystis* infection is suspected, vigorous early attempts at diagnosis and therapy are strongly recommended.

CASE A–6

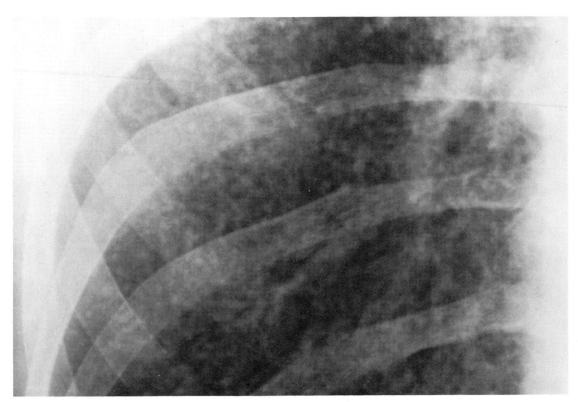

Figure A–6 Close-up

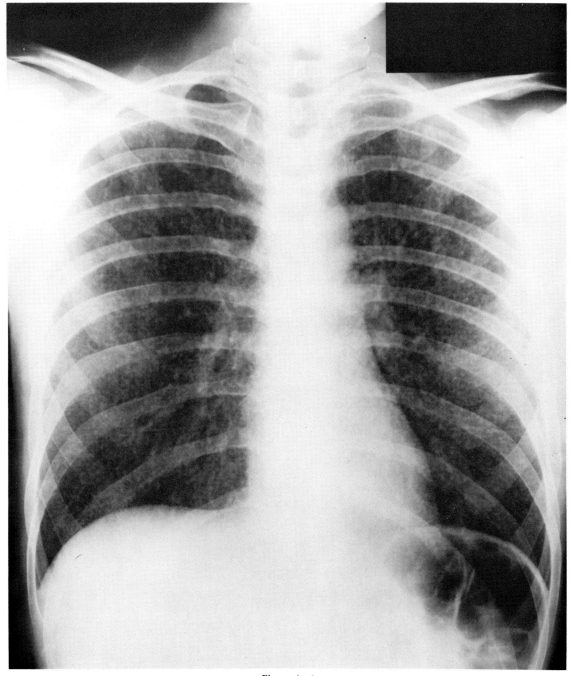

Figure A–6

Case A–6. This patient was a 28 year old white male who presented with increasing dyspnea, cough, weight loss, and fatigue. He had been under treatment with multiple drugs for stage 4B Hodgkin's disease. Therapy consisted of 1 week of bleomycin followed by 2 weeks of Cytoxan, prednisone, and procarbazine. There had been no radiation therapy or recent transfusion. Is the new chest disease caused by

1. the known neoplasm
2. a drug reaction
3. opportunistic infection

DISCUSSION, CASE A–6

Widespread pulmonary lymphoma is unlikely because the nodules are quite small, very numerous, and virtually identical in size. A diffuse granulomatous infection is the best possibility, as neither a drug reaction nor any other infection is likely to cause multiple small nodules. Although miliary tuberculosis is a possibility, the lesions are larger than expected for that disease. Open lung biopsy revealed coccidioidomycosis. One should note that the multiple nodules are very compatible with a diffuse granulomatous reaction. This is not an uncommon appearance of coccidioidomycosis in the immunosuppressed patient but is rarely, if ever, seen in the normal host. Although in the desert in the southwestern United States, coccidioidomycosis is a relatively common opportunistic invader, in other areas other fungi must be considered.

CASE A–7 _____

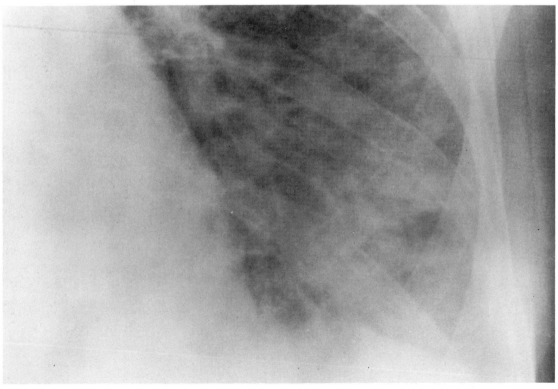

Figure A–7 Close-up

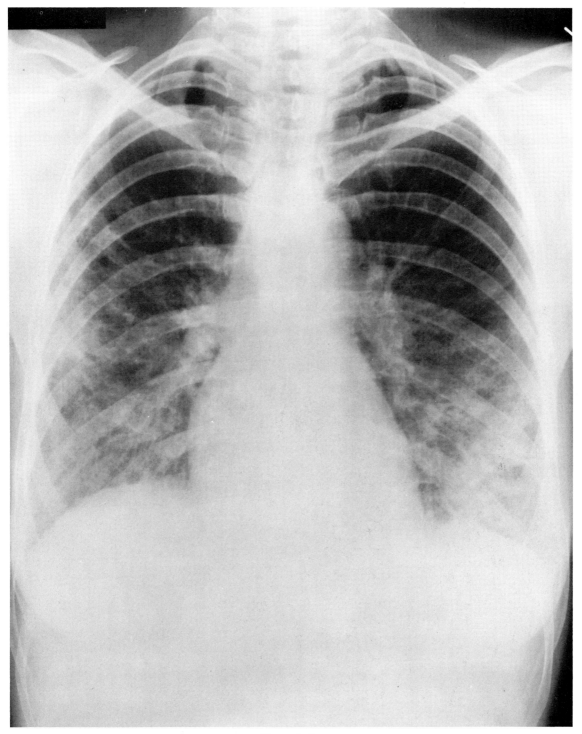

Figure A–7

Case A–7. This patient was a 55 year old white male with a known carcinoma of the anus on bleomycin therapy, who presented with increasing dyspnea and a nonproductive cough. The patient had received no recent blood transfusions. Is the new chest disease caused by

1. the known neoplasm
2. a drug reaction
3. opportunistic infection

DISCUSSION, CASE A-7

In this case the differential diagnosis involves all three possibilities, as a drug reaction, a diffuse opportunistic infection, and lymphangitic spread of the patient's known neoplasm must be considered. However, lymphangitic spread is much less likely because of the site of the primary neoplasm, the absence of any pulmonary hematogenous nodules or lymphadenopathy, and the asymmetry of the pulmonary disease. Would you choose an opportunistic infection or a reaction to bleomycin therapy? The peripheral location of much of the parenchymal disease suggests infection, while the bilaterality of the process is more in favor of a reaction to bleomycin. In this type of case an early biopsy to rule out infection is recommended. (Which method of biopsy is best is controversial and will not be discussed here.)

Within 6 weeks the pulmonary parenchymal reaction had completely cleared but the patient succumbed 6 months later to bone marrow hypoplasia and to renal, cardiac, and pulmonary failure. The multiple organ system failure found at autopsy strongly suggested that the bleomycin was the probable cause of the pulmonary disease 6 months before as well as the cause of death.

CASE A-8

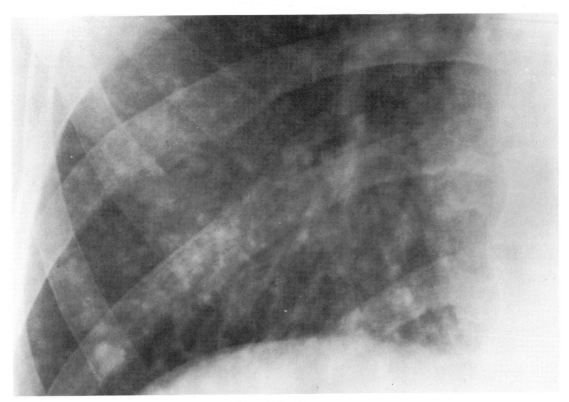

Figure A–8 Close-up

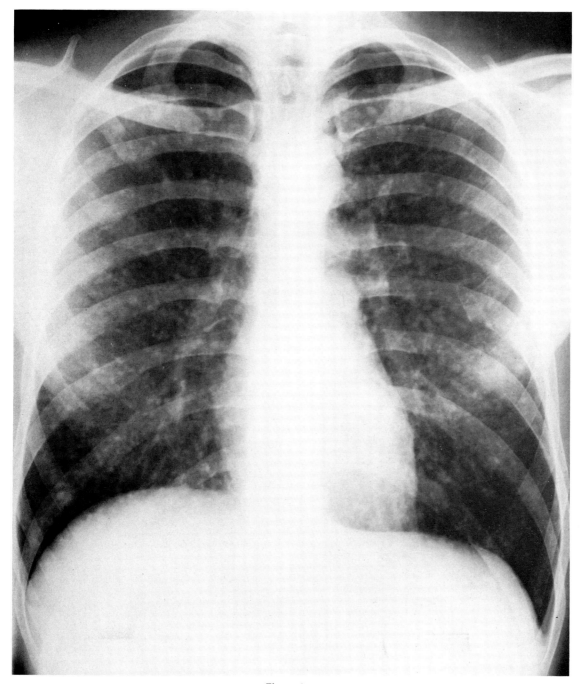

Figure A–8

Case A–8. This was a 32 year old white male who was under therapy with DTIC (dimethyltriazenoimidazole carboxamide) and BCNU (bischloronitrosourea) for known melanoma. He complained only of moderate malaise and fatigue. Is the new chest disease caused by

1. the known neoplasm
2. a drug reaction
3. opportunistic infection

DISCUSSION, CASE A–8

The multiple small nodules limit the differential diagnosis to the hematogenous spread of the patient's known melanoma or an opportunistic granulomatous infection. Which would you choose? If you chose an opportunistic granulomatous infection, you didn't look closely enough. Compare the close-up of this patient with Figure A–6 close-up. In this case the multiple nodules are relatively well circumscribed and show a variation in size, in contrast to those in the patient with diffuse coccidioidomycosis. The patient eventually succumbed to widespread hematogenous metastases.

CASE A–9 _____

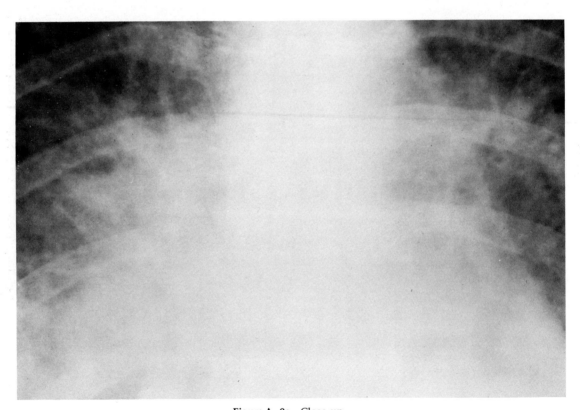

Figure A–9a   Close-up

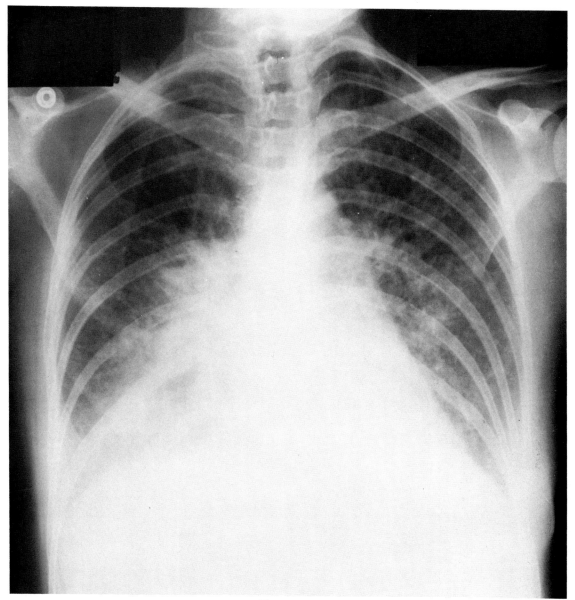

Figure A–9a

Case A–9a. This patient was a 44 year old white female who presented with acute dyspnea. She had had a right mastectomy for carcinoma of the breast approximately 2 years earlier and had been maintained on Adriamycin therapy. Is the new chest disease caused by

1. the known neoplasm
2. a drug reaction
3. opportunistic infection

A radiograph of this patient made 2 days later is on the next page (Fig. A–9b).

CASE A–9 *CONTINUED*

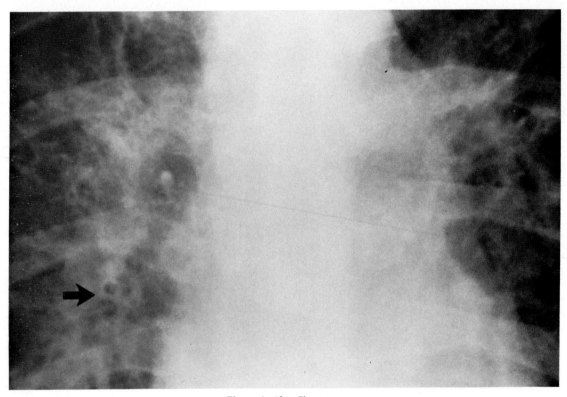

Figure A–9b   Close-up

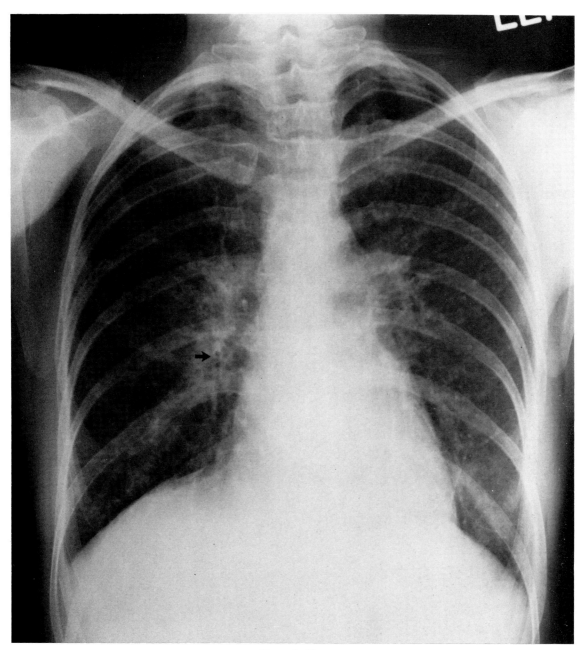

Figure A–9b

Case A–9b. This is the same patient shown in Figure A–9a following 2 days of bed rest and diuresis. The initial radiograph is certainly compatible with pulmonary edema, but why should this 44 year old woman suffer heart failure?

In Figure A–9b it is noteworthy that although much of the fluid has been cleared from the lungs, interstitial edema remains and can be recognized by the edematous peribronchial soft tissues about each hilum (arrow). One should also be aware that the patient may have presented several days before she did with the very same picture of interstitial pulmonary edema seen here.

DISCUSSION, CASE A–9

In this case the diagnosis certainly cannot be made from the radiographs alone. The patient was in congestive heart failure, which is a well-known sequela of Adriamycin therapy. As far as the differential diagnosis is concerned, lymphangitic spread of the patient's known neoplasm would have been a possibility, and an opportunistic infection could not have been entirely excluded. However, the central and symmetric appearance makes infection a less likely possibility. The patient was treated with diuresis and bed rest, and much of the pulmonary edema had cleared in 2 days (Fig. A—9b).

CASE A–10

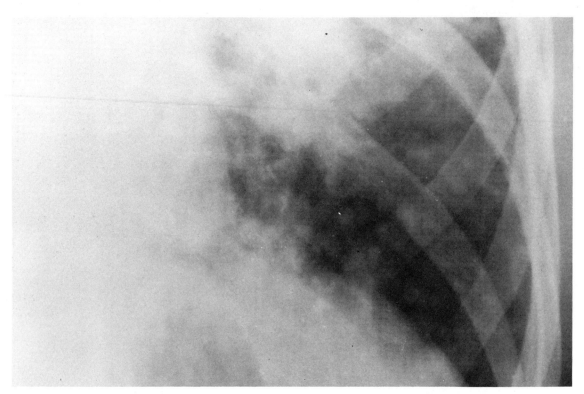

Figure A–10   Close-up

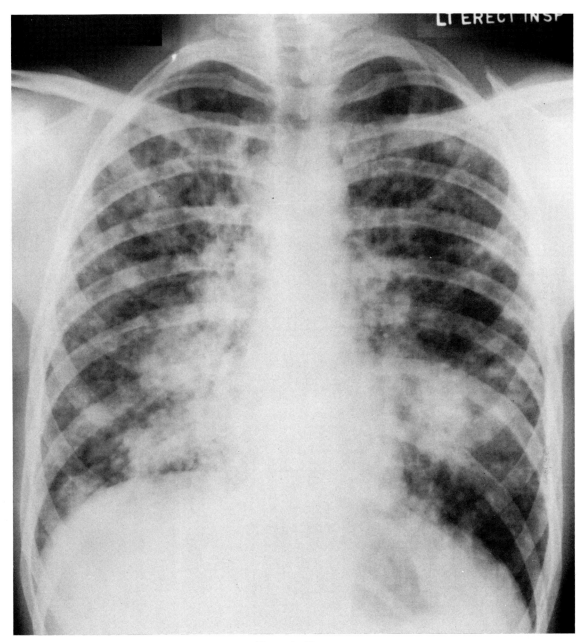

Figure A–10

Case A–10. This patient was a 16 year old white male who presented with a rash, fever, cough, and shortness of breath. The patient was known to have Hodgkin's disease and was treated with prednisone and Cytoxan but had been lost to follow-up for the 6 months prior to admission. Several weeks prior to admission the patient was vaccinated against smallpox in the usual fashion by a physician who did not know of the lymphoma. Is the new chest disease caused by

1. the known neoplasm
2. a drug reaction
3. opportunistic infection

DISCUSSION, CASE A–10

In this case the differential diagnosis lies between opportunistic infection and the patient's known lymphoma. Which would you choose? If you selected a diffuse vaccinia pneumonia, you've gone right down the garden path. The history of a vaccination in a patient who was probably immunosuppressed is enticing; however, close observation of the radiograph will reveal not only lymphadenopathy but multiple pulmonary nodules that are relatively well circumscribed and show a considerable variation in size. The patient died a short time later, and his lungs were found to be totally involved with Hodgkin's disease.

(In an immunosuppressed patient fever is frequently absent despite infection but is, of course, often present in lymphoma without infection. Fever is not a highly reliable piece of clinical information in the immunosuppressed patient.)

CASE A–11

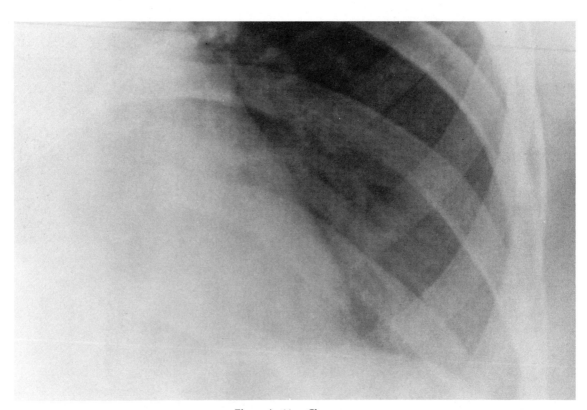

Figure A–11a   Close-up

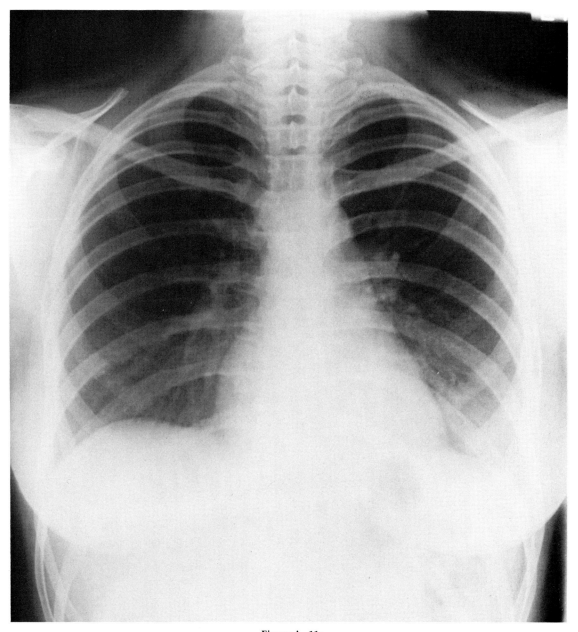

Figure A–11a

Case A–11a. This 15 year old white female presented with dyspnea, lethargy, fever, and chills. She also had otitis externa and monilial pharyngitis. The patient had been under therapy for non-Hodgkin's lymphoma with multiple agents, most recently Cytoxan, Velban, and prednisone. In the past she had also taken vincristine, bleomycin, and Adriamycin. Is the new chest disease caused by

1. the known neoplasm
2. a drug reaction
3. opportunistic infection

See Figures A–11b and A–11c on the next two pages.

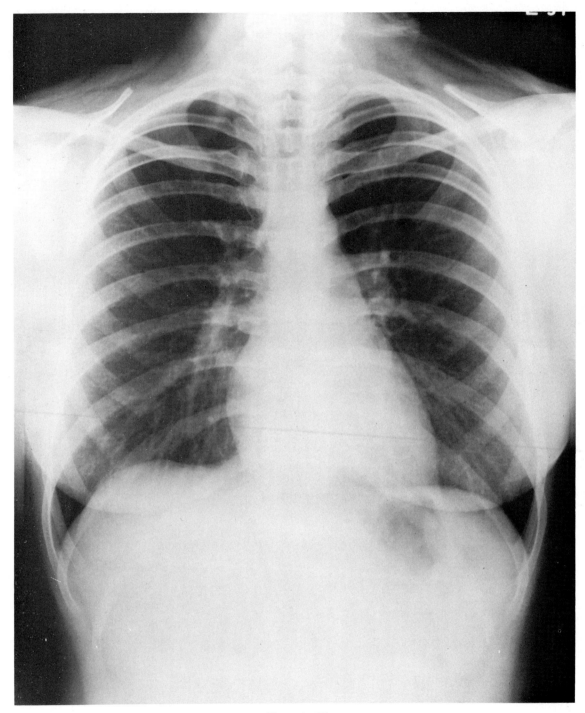

Figure A–11b

Case A–11b. This is the same patient as in Figure A–11a when she was asymptomatic, several months before her last admission.

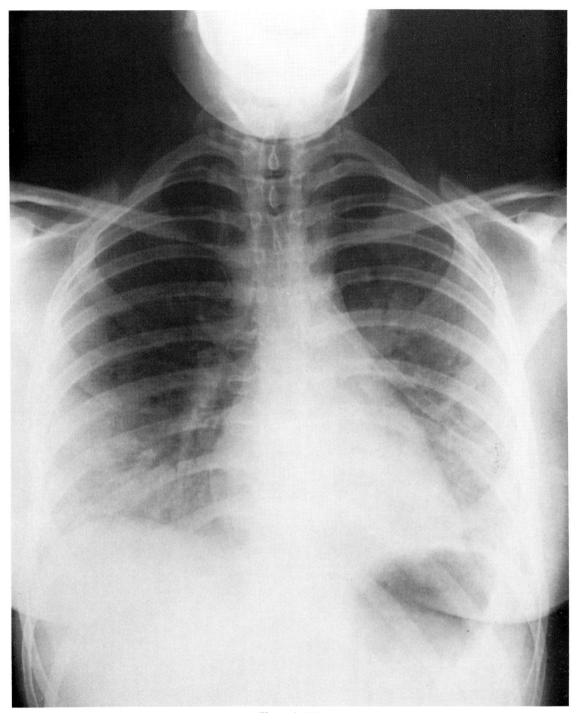

Figure A–11c

Case A–11c. This is the same patient as in Figures A–11a and A–11b 8 days following admission. She was suffering from a marked increase in dyspnea.

DISCUSSION, CASE A–11

Once again the question is whether the chest radiograph is normal or abnormal. The depth of the patient's inspiration is much greater in Figure A–11b than it is in Figure A–11a. However, one should not automatically assume that this is an error on the part of the technologist. Patients with diffuse interstitial disease are often unable to take a deep breath. This phenomenon is secondary to diminished pulmonary compliance and may also be seen with diffuse interstitial hydrostatic pulmonary edema.

The diffuse interstitial process, which later also involves the alveolar space(s) (Fig. A–11b), is due to either a drug reaction or a diffuse infection. The greater involvement of the peripheral portions of the lungs again suggests that an infection is most likely. While a viral etiology must be considered, in this type of patient *Pneumocystis carinii* should be the primary diagnosis, as far as an opportunistic invader is concerned. Even if the patient eventually proves to have a parenchymal reaction to drug therapy, a vigorous attempt to diagnose and treat *Pneumocystis carinii* pneumonia must be made as early as possible. This patient eventually succumbed to *Pneumocystis carinii* pneumonia as well as to a massive intracerebral hemorrhage.

CASE A–12

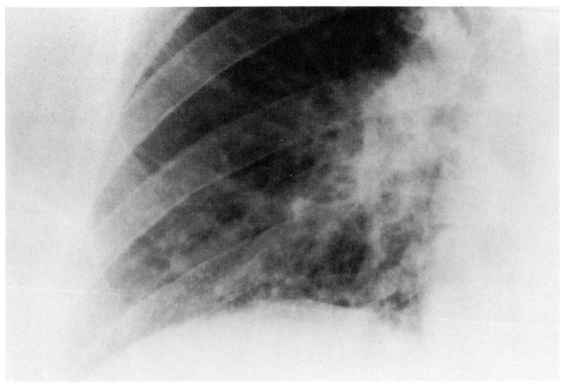

Figure A–12a   Close-up

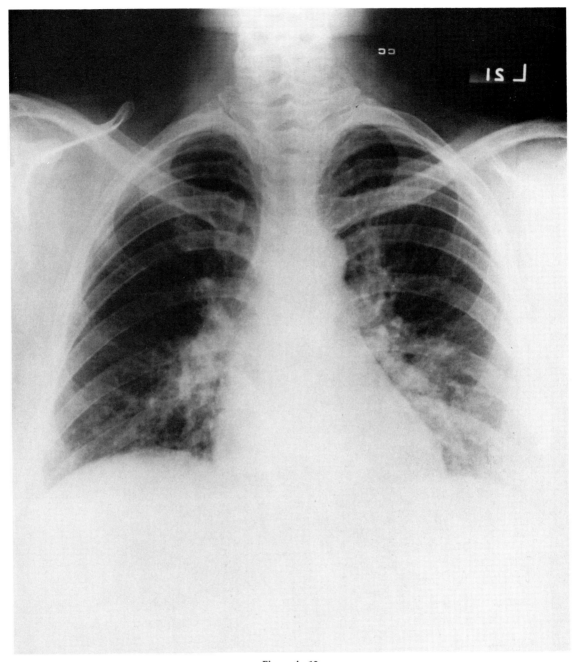

Figure A–12a

Case A–12a. This patient was a 40 year old white female who presented with anorexia, weight loss, and pelvic pain. She had a known endometrial carcinoma and was taking only pain medication. Is the new chest disease caused by

1. the neoplasm itself
2. opportunistic infection

After you have made your decision as to the probable diagnosis turn the page for a radiograph of the same patient made 4 months later.

CASE A–12 *CONTINUED*

Did you note the nodular densities in the right lower lobe? They are fairly well marginated and show a considerable variation in size and are compatible with hematogenous metastases from the patient's known carcinoma. They are probably present in the left lower lobe as well but are partially obscured by another process. What process do you think may be obscuring them?

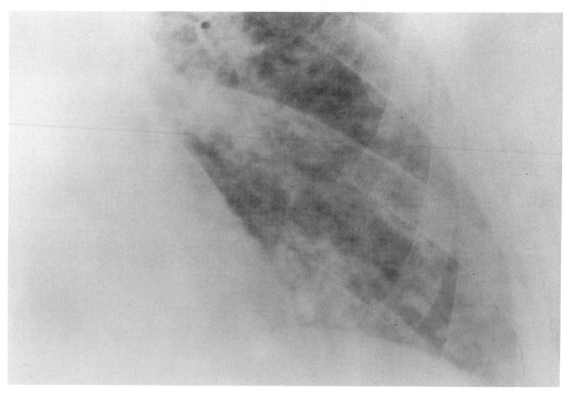

Figure A–12b   Close-up

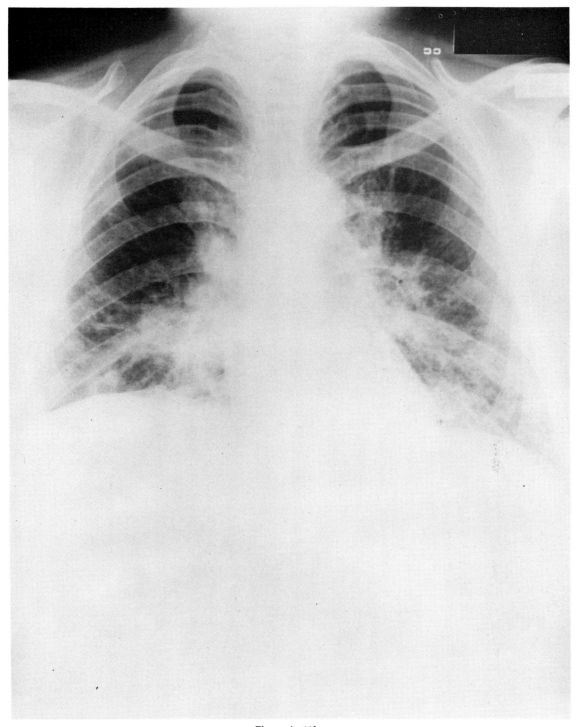

Figure A-12b

Case A-12b. This is the same patient as shown in Figure A-12a 4 months later. At this time she was complaining of considerable abdominal pain, nausea, and vomiting. She was taking no chemotherapeutic agents and had not had a blood transfusion or radiation therapy to the chest. Do you think the new chest disease is caused by

1. the neoplasm itself
2. opportunistic infection

DISCUSSION, CASE A-12

The radiograph made 4 months later shows increased disease in both lower lobes, most of which is secondary to lymphangitic spread of carcinoma. The metastatic nodules are larger. Janower and Blennerhassett[6] have shown that most lymphangitic spread of carcinoma in the lung emanates from originally hematogenous foci. Close observation of many cases of lymphangitic spread of carcinoma in the lung will enable one to see the underlying hematogenous nodules. Superimposed infection is difficult to exclude, particularly on the right side, but if present it would be expected to be more peripheral than central.

CASE A-13

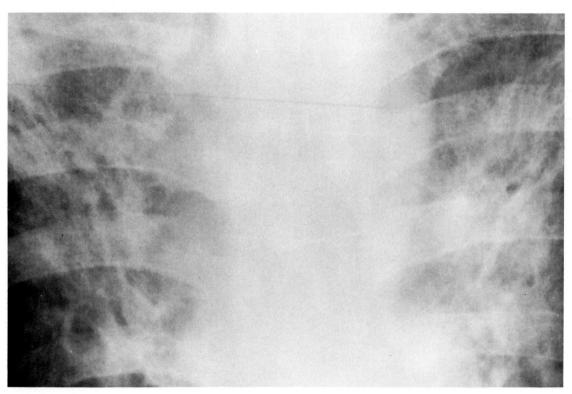

Figure A-13 Close-up

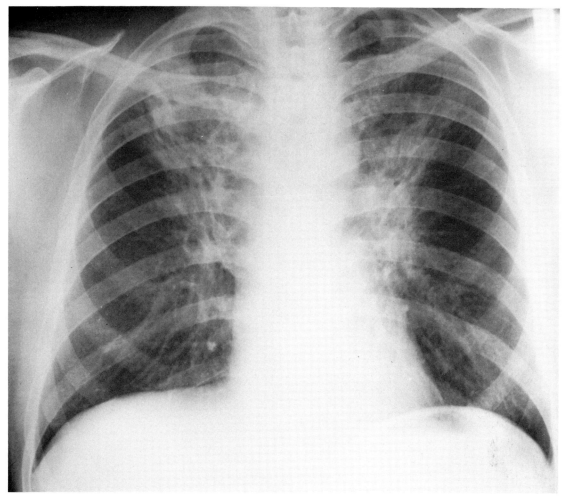

Figure A–13

Case A–13. This patient was a 49 year old white male who presented with a severe nonproductive cough. He had been under care for Hodgkin's disease discovered 6 months earlier. What do you think is the cause of his current pulmonary parenchymal disease? (This case courtesy of Edwin S. Roth, M.D., Tucson, Arizona.)

DISCUSSION, CASE A–13

As with most cases of radiation pneumonitis or fibrosis, the margins of the disease are rather sharply defined. This margination is caused by the shape of the portal used in radiation therapy. Differential diagnosis is not usually a problem, but recurrence of the patient's known neoplasm, either within the treated field or adjacent to it, must always be given consideration.

CASE A–14 _____

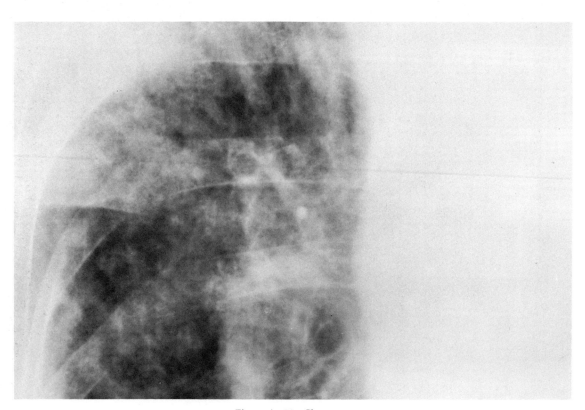

Figure A–14   Close-up

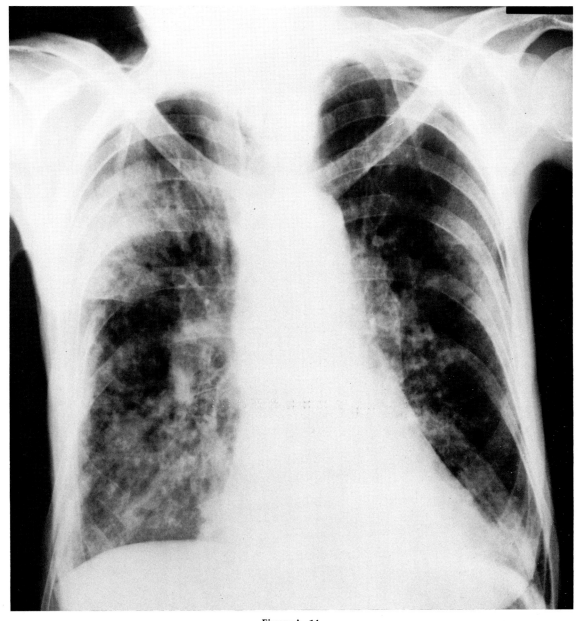

Figure A-14

Case A-14.   This patient was a 75 year old white female who presented with fever and cough. She had had non-Hodgkin's lymphoma for approximately 6 years and had been treated over the years with radiation therapy to multiple sites and with various courses of chemotherapy. Her last course of chemotherapy was 4 weeks of Adriamycin, which terminated 2 months before the current admission. There was no recent blood transfusion. Is the new chest disease caused by

1. the known neoplasm
2. a drug reaction
3. opportunistic infection
4. radiation reaction

DISCUSSION, CASE A–14

This case is a difficult one, as there may be two diseases present in the lungs. One is an alveolar filling process in the right upper lobe and the other, is multinodular disease in both lungs but primarily on the right side. The homogeneous appearance and the peripheral location of the process in the right upper lobe strongly suggest an infection, probably bacterial. The nodular component is secondary to either the patient's known lymphoma or a second opportunistic infection. Both klebsiella and *Candida albicans* were cultured from this patient's sputum. She succumbed to these infections approximately 1 week after the radiograph was made. No lymphoma was present in her lungs.

CASE A–15 _____

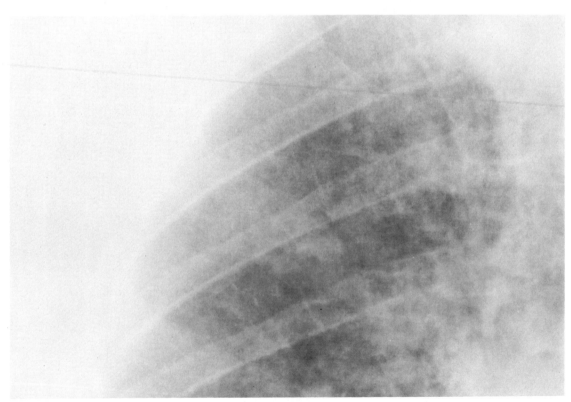

Figure A–15a   Close-up

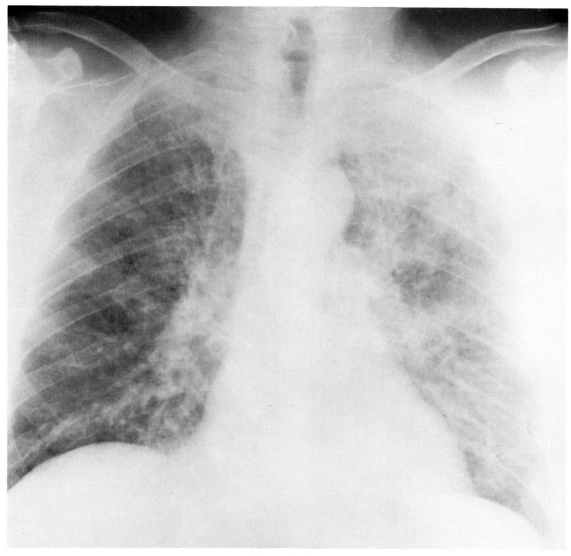

Figure A–15a

Case A–15a. This patient was a 63 year old white male who presented with fever, anemia, and a marked leukopenia. He was under therapy for acute myelogenous leukemia with DOAP (daunomycin, vincristine (Oncovin), arabinoside, and prednisone). He was transfused several times on the second and third hospital days with whole blood and packed cells. Because of the severe leukopenia he was treated with multiple antibiotics. On the fourth hosptial day he became dyspneic, and the radiograph seen here was made. The chest radiograph on admission was within normal limits. Is the new chest disease caused by

1. known neoplasm
2. a drug reaction
3. opportunistic infection
4. transfusion reaction

After you have evaluated this radiograph, turn the page for additional examinations of the same patient.

CASE A–15 *CONTINUED*

This type of disease is difficult to diagnose because of the multiple possibilities. The central and relatively symmetric pulmonary pattern is compatible with a drug reaction, a transfusion reaction, and congestive heart failure. Because of the marked leukocyte depletion, widespread infection cannot be excluded.

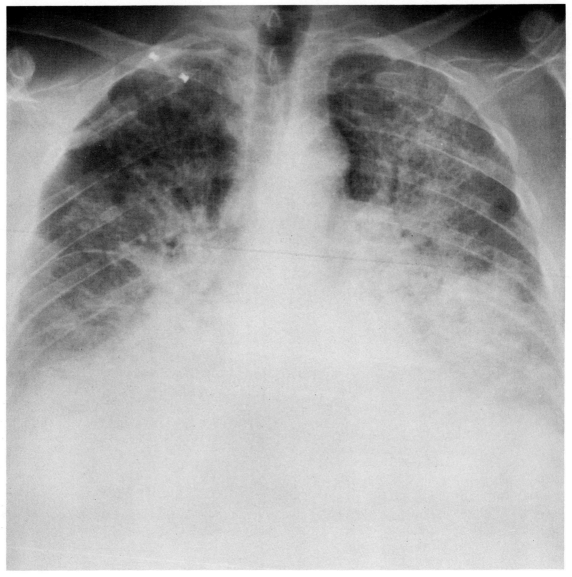

Figure A–15b

Case A–15b. This is the same patient shown in Figure A–15a. By the eighth hospital day the bilateral parenchymal process had become much more severe with considerable airspace filling in both lungs.

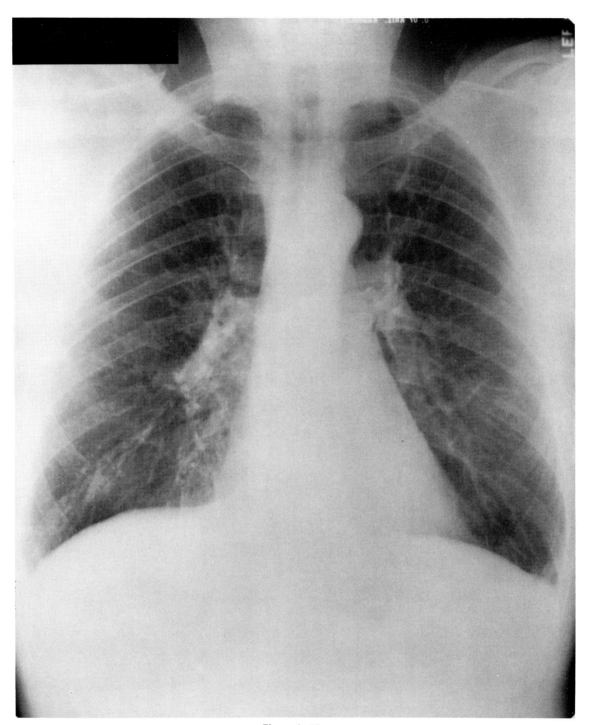

Figure A–15c

Case A–15c. This is the same patient shown in Figures A–15a and A–15b. By the fifteenth hospital day the patient was almost completely well and ready for discharge. What is the best diagnosis?

DISCUSSION, CASE A–15

This central and symmetric nature of the pulmonary disease on both radiographs is the clue to the diagnosis. As time progressed a transfusion reaction became a less likely possibility, and, although the patient did have a urinary tract infection, multiple blood cultures were negative. The roentgen picture is highly compatible with congestive heart failure, and the patient was taking a cardiotoxic drug, daunomycin. Treatment with diuretics resulted in diuresis and rapid clinical improvement (Fig. A–15c).

CASE A–16

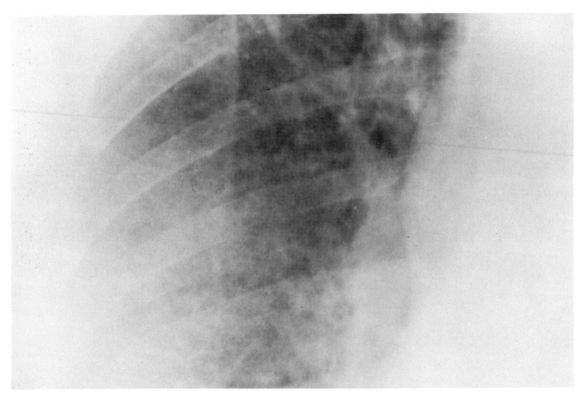

Figure A–16a   Close-up

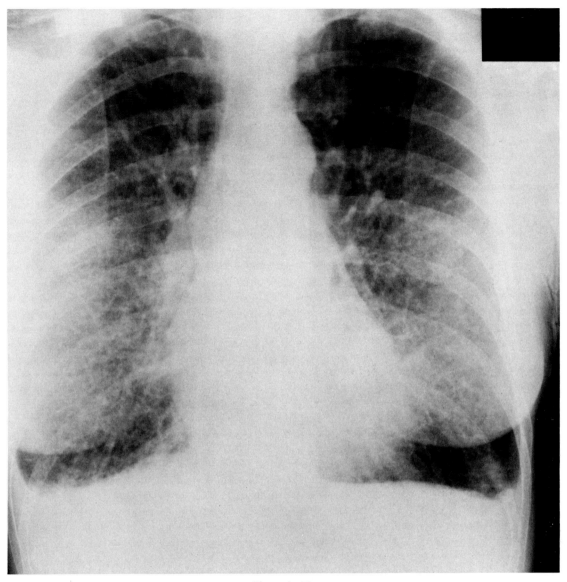

Figure A–16a

Case A–16a. This patient was a 62 year old white female who had acute myelocytic leukemia, and at the time of the current radiograph she had severe leukocyte depletion and was febrile. She had been treated during the previous month with multiple blood transfusions and antibiotics. Treatment with multiple chemotherapeutic agents and prednisone was begun 2 weeks before this radiograph was made. What do you think is responsible for the patient's current chest disease?

1. the known neoplasm
2. a drug reaction
3. opportunistic infection
4. blood transfusion

There is an additional radiographic examination of this patient on the next page.

CASE A–16 *CONTINUED*

If you think the patient might have had *Pneumocystis carinii* pneumonitis, your thinking corresponds with ours at that time. Septra was added to the regimen of antibiotics and amphotericin B that the patient was already on. Although she had had three blood transfusions within the 2 days prior to this radiograph, the interstitial nature of the disease and the pleural effusions indicated that this was not a transfusion reaction. Leukemic infiltrations in the lung are very rare, but owing to platelet depletion or thrombocytopenia, leukemia can cause pulmonary hemorrhage. This possibility could not be eliminated and may have been present at that time, although there was no hemoptysis. A drug reaction was the third viable possibility, but in that case pleural effusions would not have been expected.

CASE A–16 _____

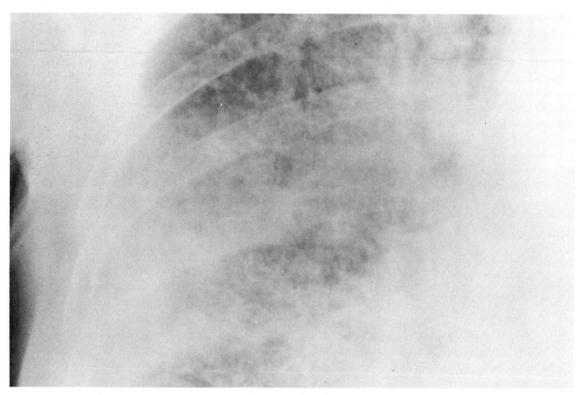

Figure A–16b   Close-up

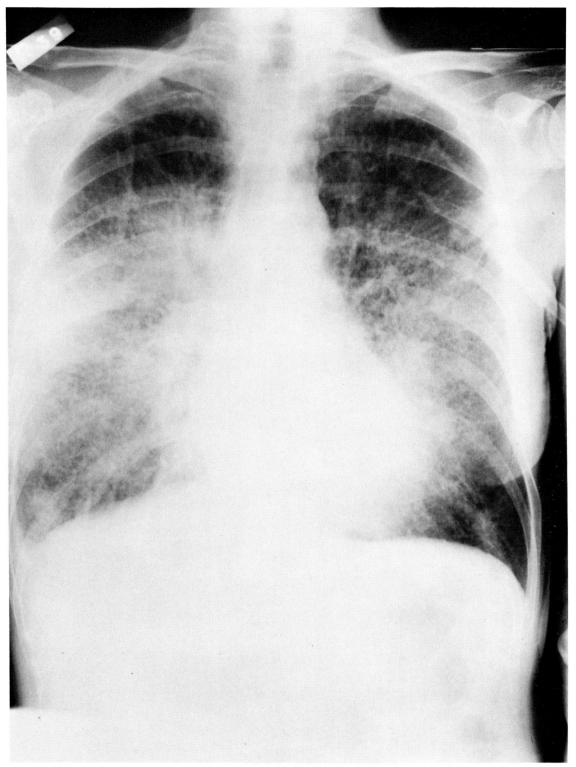

Figure A–16b

Case A–16b. This is the same patient shown in Figure A–16a 2 weeks later. Despite chemotherapy, antibiotics, and blood transfusions, the patient's condition continued to deteriorate, and the radiographic picture noted here gradually developed. What is your first choice of diagnosis at this time?

DISCUSSION, CASE A–16

The peripheral alveolar nature of the process now present on the right side, which can barely be seen on the earlier radiograph, strongly suggests that infection now dominates (Fig. A–16b). While the possibility of a reaction to one of the chemotherapeutic agents could not be entirely eliminated, and hemorrhage secondary to the patient's known leukemia was even more difficult to eliminate, infection was the most likely possibility. *Aspergillus fumigatus* was cultured from the patient's sputum, although she had been placed on an amphotericin B regimen several weeks before. She succumbed several days later, and autopsy revealed widespread pulmonary aspergillosis as well as hemorrhage.

CASE A–17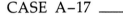

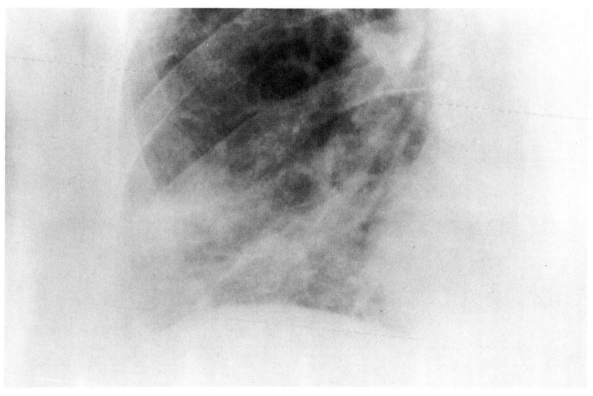

Figure A–17 Close-up

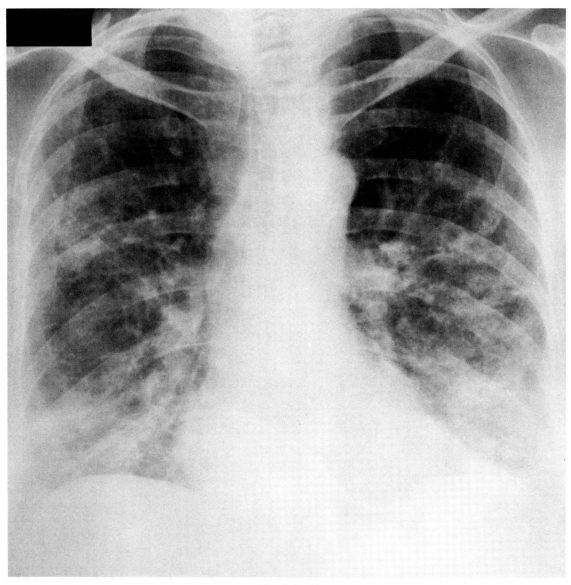

Figure A–17

Case A–17. This patient was a 63 year old white female who presented with recurrent fever, fatigue, weakness, and dyspnea. She had been treated for several years for chronic lymphocytic leukemia with many different chemotherapeutic regimens and radiation therapy to multiple sites. The drugs used included chlorambucil (Leukeran), Cytoxan, bleomycin, Adriamycin, vincristine, and prednisone. The white blood cell count was over 300,000, but 98 per cent of these cells were lymphocytes. The patient was not anemic, and there had been no recent blood transfusions. Do you think the new chest disease is caused by

    1. the known neoplasm
    2. a drug reaction
    3. opportunistic infection

DISCUSSION, CASE A–17

The patient's neoplasm would be a most unlikely cause of the bilateral parenchymal infiltrations, even if one considers the possibility of intrapulmonary hemorrhage secondary to platelet depletion or thrombocytopenia. There are two viable possibilities, a reaction to one of the drugs or an opportunistic infection. Which would you choose?

A new infection in this immunosuppressed patient is the correct choice. However, the appearance of the radiograph is generally inadequate to determine the microbiological diagnosis. In this case the picture is compatible with a bacterial, viral, or *Pneumocystis carinii* infection, and aspergillosis cannot be excluded. Despite all supportive measures, this patient succumbed approximately 2 weeks later, and autopsy revealed severe active interstitial pneumonitis secondary to herpes simplex.

CASE A–18 _____

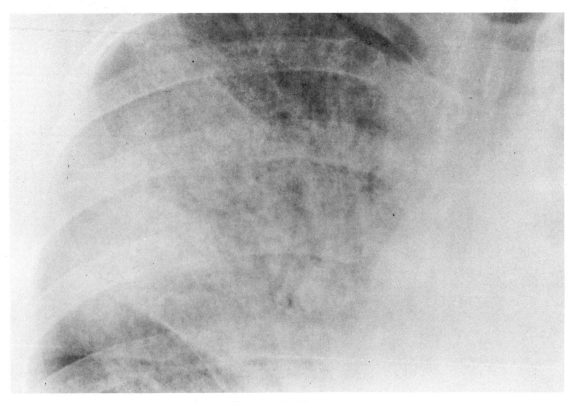

Figure A–18   Close-up

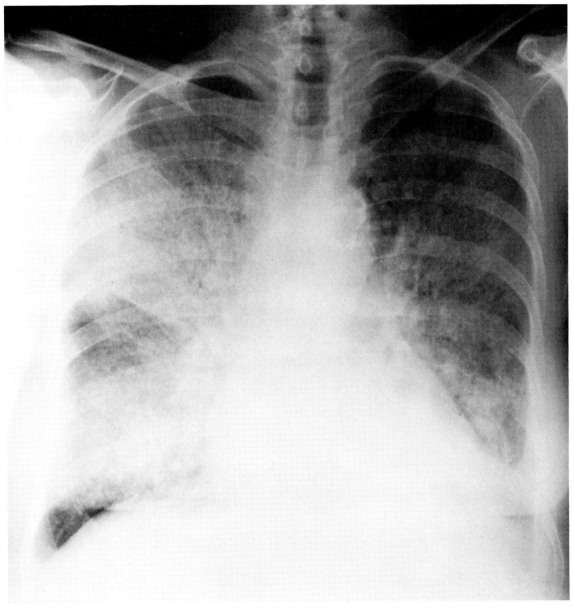

Figure A–18

Case A–18. This patient is a 61 year old white female who at the time of the radiograph had considerable dyspnea and a nonproductive cough. She was admitted to the hospital for the induction of chemotherapy 17 days before the radiograph was made, with the diagnosis of acute myelogenous leukemia. Therapy consisted of vincristine, Adriamycin, Ara-C, and prednisone. She tolerated this therapy well; however, it resulted in pancytopenia and fever with a white blood cell count of less than 1000 for the remainder of her hospital course. For this she required packed red blood cell, platelet, and leukocyte transfusions. She developed severe dyspnea and hypoxia just before the radiograph presented here was made. Chest radiographs made on admission and 6 days later were both normal. What do you think is the cause of the sudden onset of diffuse pulmonary disease?

DISCUSSION, CASE A–18

This is a difficult case with multiple possibilities. The differential diagnosis lies between a transfusion reaction, a drug reaction, pulmonary hemorrhage, and an opportunistic infection, most likely *Pneumocystis carinii*. At autopsy there was a diffuse inflammatory reaction in the interstitium of each lung, but no organism — bacteria, fungi, viruses, or pneumocystis — could be detected. The most likely diagnosis, although it cannot be proved is a leukocyte-mediated transfusion reaction. There was no hemorrhage found in the lungs at autopsy, and because of the time relationships a drug reaction is a less likely possibility. The role of the radiologist in such a case is to make the clinician aware of the various possibilities, even though a definitive single diagnosis cannot be made.

REFERENCES

1. Blank, N., Castellino, R. A., and Shah, V.: Radiographic aspects of pulmonary infection in patients with altered immunity. Radiol. Clin. North Am., 11(1):175–190, 1973.
2. Bragg, D. G., and Janis, B.: The radiographic manifestations of pulmonary opportunistic infections. Radiol. Clin. North Am., 11(2):357, 1973.
3. Brettner, A., Heitzman, R., and Woodin, W.: Pulmonary complications of drug therapy. Radiology, 96:31–38, 1970.
4. Fraser, R. G., and Paré, J. A. P.: Diagnosis of Diseases of the Chest, 2nd ed. Philadelphia, W. B. Saunders Co., 1977.
5. Golde, D. W., Drew, W. L., Klein, H. Z., et al.: Occult pulmonary haemorrhage in leukaemia. Br. Med. J., 2:166–169, 1975.
6. Janower, M., and Blennerhassett, J.: Lymphangitic spread of metastatic cancer to the lung. Radiology, 101:267–273, 1971.
7. Libshitz, H. I., and Southard, M. E.: Complications of radiation therapy: The thorax. Semin. Roentgenol., 9:41–49, 1974.
8. Ward, H. N.: Pulmonary infiltrates associated with leukoagglutinin transfusion reactions. Ann. Intern. Med., 73:689–694, 1970.
9. Webb, W. R., Gamsu, G., Rohlfing, B. M., et al.: Pulmonary complications of renal transplantation: A survey of patients treated by low-dose immunosuppression. Radiology, 126:1–8, 1978
10. Williams, D. M., Krick, J. A., and Remington, J. S.: Pulmonary infection in the compromised host. In Murray, J. F. (ed.): Lung Disease — State of the Art 1975–1976. New York, American Lung Association, 1977, pp. 131–201.
11. Zornoza, J., Goldman, A. M., Wallace, S., et al.: Radiologic features of gram-negative pneumonias in the neutropenic patient. Am. J. Roentgenol., 127:989–996, 1976.

Section B

If the patient is not known to be immunosuppressed, then the second question one should ask is whether the disease is *multinodular*.

Decision 1. One should always consider the acutely ill patient first. If multiple pulmonary nodules are present they may be caused by:

a. the nodular form of pulmonary edema
b. an acute viral infection
c. septic emboli

If a patient with significant chronic obstructive pulmonary disease suffers left heart failure, there is often an unusual pattern of pulmonary edema. One of these patterns is multinodular and will be discussed more fully in another section. Rarely, pulmonary edema may appear nodular in patients without known obstructive airways disease, and although various theories have been put forth, a definitive explanation is not known. A multinodular acute viral infection is usually secondary to varicella, which although uncommon, must be kept in mind, particularly with individuals who may not have been exposed in childhood. Septic embolization produces pulmonary nodules with surrounding pneumonitis; these cavitate rapidly and are usually not difficult to diagnose because the patient most often has an obvious infection elsewhere.

Decision 2. Although some patients with miliary tuberculosis present with acute illness, most are subacutely or chronically ill and will be considered in Decision 2, which asks whether the nodules represent granulomata. (It is advantageous to consider all multiple nodular masses to be in the multinodular category whether there are a few large masses or innumerable tiny nodules.) If the nodules are small granulomata rather than metastases, they will be approximately the same in size, 1 to 3 millimeters in diameter, and the margins of each nodule will be irregular. If this is the case, the four most common granulomatous processes should be considered:

1. miliary tuberculosis
2. sarcoidosis
3. silicosis (pneumoconiosis)
4. fungal infection

Miliary tuberculosis should always be the primary consideration because it is life-threatening, curable, and easily missed. The following are several important points that tend to differentiate the four common granulomatous nodular diseases:

1. Miliary tuberculosis
   a. The nodules are usually very small but often are superimposed radiographically.
   b. The nodules are usually evenly and widely distributed.
   c. Reinfection tuberculosis may well be present.
   d. The patient may present with tuberculous meningitis.
2. Sarcoidosis
   a. The nodules are usually more central than peripheral, and the apices and bases of the lungs are often spared.
   b. Lymphadenopathy is present in about 75 per cent of patients who have thoracic sarcoidosis. The typical appearance is bilat-

eral hilar lymphadenopathy (of the bronchial lymph nodes) or bilateral hilar and right paratracheal lymphadenopathy (Garland's Triad).

   c. The granulomata may have a linear appearance.

   d. Complications of sarcoidosis that may be seen early in the disease usually consist of superimposed fibrosis and cyst formation. Occasionally fibrotic masses, cavitation, and mycetomata develop.

3. Silicosis (pneumoconiosis)

   a. The nodules usually favor the upper lobes.

   b. Moderate lymphadenopathy may be present— a rim type of calcification is typical.

   c. Conglomerate masses are often present and are usually in the upper lobes and relatively symmetric.

   d. Associated fibrosis and compensatory hyperaeration is often present.

4. Fungal infection

In this category the most common fungal infection is the multinodular form of histoplasmosis.

Decision 3. If the multiple nodules are not granulomatous, then Decision 3 must be whether they could be metastatic. Multiple very small nodules may be seen in metastatic carcinoma of the breast, in carcinoma of the thyroid, in melanoma, and less commonly, but possibly, in any neoplasm. To be considered metastatic, nodules should meet the two criteria mentioned previously in Section A.

   a. The nodules should vary considerably in size.

   b. The margins of each nodule should be relatively smooth.

Decision 4. At this point in the differential diagnosis of multiple nodules, alveolar cell carcinoma must be considered. Most alveolar cell carcinomas present as a solitary mass. In a significant percentage of cases, however, the presentation is one of multiple small nodules widely distributed throughout the chest, but the radiograph is still distinctive because the solitary mass is almost always present as well. The nodules are quite small and are located in the alveolar spaces rather than in the interstitium. The exact location of the nodules is exceedingly difficult to determine radiographically.

Although the initial presentation of diffuse pulmonary lymphoma is almost invariably marked by mediastinal or hilar lymphadenopathy, or both, occasionally a patient initially presents with diffuse ill-defined pulmonary nodules without lymphadenopathy. The most common lymphoma to present in this fashion is the diffuse histiocytic variety.

Decision 5. Finally, Decision 5, the uncommon granulomatous diseases, must be considered:

1. Rheumatoid nodules

   a. The relatively few nodules are smoother in outline than other granulomata.

   b. The nodules frequently cavitate.

   c. Caplan's syndrome may be present.

   d. Rheumatoid arthritis is usually but not always well established.

2. Wegener's granulomatosis

   a. The nodules or granulomatous masses are usually quite large, relatively few in number, and grossly irregular in outline.

   b. These granulomatous masses frequently cavitate.

   c. The paranasal sinuses and kidneys are involved unless the limited form of Wegener's disease is present.

3. Histiocytosis X (eosinophilic granuloma)

   a. The disease occurs in young patients.

   b. The condition is frequently associated with significant fibrosis and formation of multiple small cysts.

4. Berylliosis

   a. The appearance is usually not nodular but very finely granular.

   b. Minimal to moderate lymphadenopathy may be present.

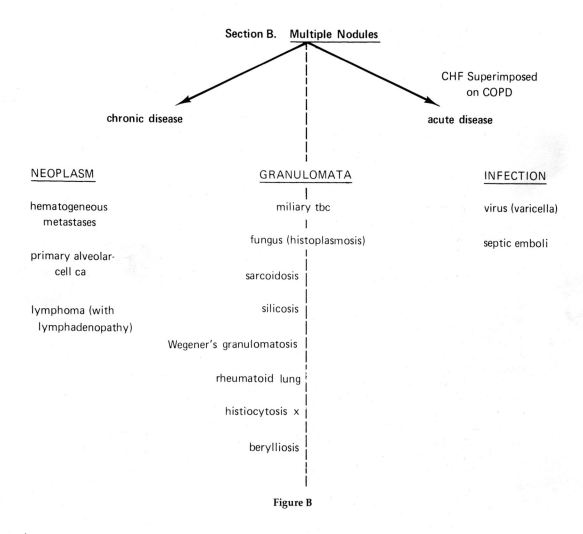

Section B.   Multiple Nodules

chronic disease

CHF Superimposed
on COPD

acute disease

NEOPLASM

hematogeneous
metastases

primary alveolar-
cell ca

lymphoma (with
lymphadenopathy)

GRANULOMATA

miliary tbc

fungus (histoplasmosis)

sarcoidosis

silicosis

Wegener's granulomatosis

rheumatoid lung

histiocytosis x

berylliosis

INFECTION

virus (varicella)

septic emboli

Figure B

CASE B–1

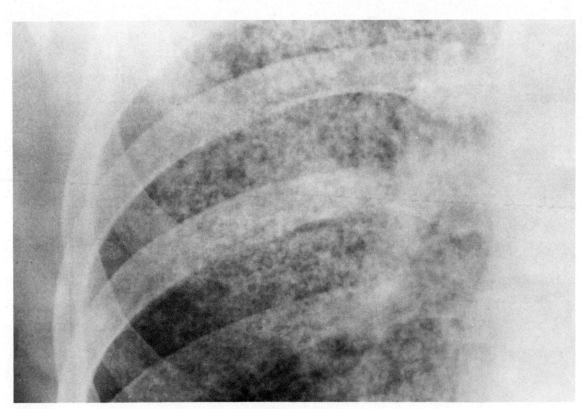

Figure B–1   Close-up

Figure B–1

Case B–1. This patient was a 33 year old white male who presented with 10 days of fever, malaise, and fatigue. He also had had a chronic cough and had lost weight for 2 months prior to admission. What is your diagnosis?

DISCUSSION, CASE B–1

Miliary tuberculosis, of course! The diagnosis is not uncommon and is too often missed. The nodules are even in size, very small except where there is radiographic conglomeration, and widely distributed throughout the chest in this patient, who is subacutely ill. In such a patient miliary tuberculosis *must* be the first consideration, and therapy should be started immediately. A number of other diseases may be included in the differential diagnosis, such as sarcoidosis, histoplasmosis, and histiocytosis X. However, the radiographic appearance in this case strongly favors miliary tuberculosis. In addition, there is good evidence of reinfection tuberculosis in the left upper lobe (arrow).

CASE B–2

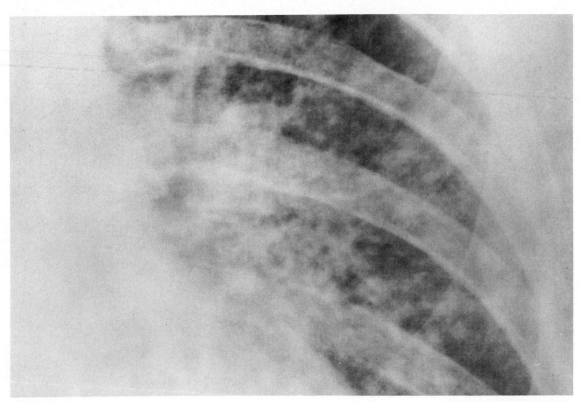

Figure B–2 Close-up

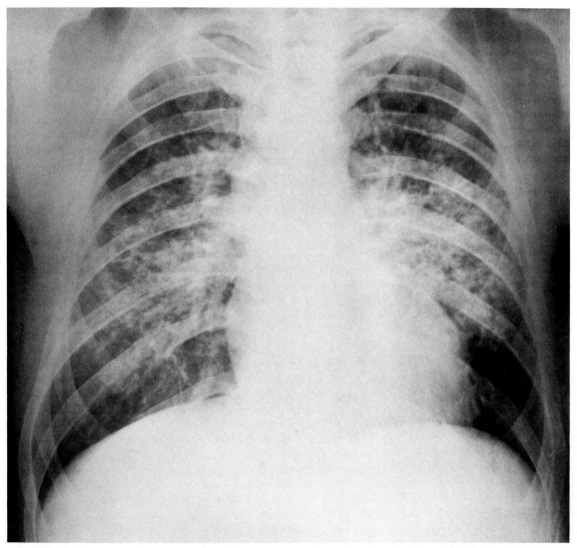

Figure B–2

Case B–2. This patient was a 25 year old black female who presented with 2 months of increasing dyspnea and a nonproductive cough. Are the nodules granulomatous? What is the best diagnosis?

DISCUSSION, CASE B–2

In making the first decision we see once again that the case clearly falls into the granulomatous category and that this case is almost pathognomonic for sarcoidosis. Not only is the disease central and relatively symmetric, sparing the apices and bases of the lungs, but some of the granulomata have a linear appearance, and lymphadenopathy is present.

CASE B–3 _____

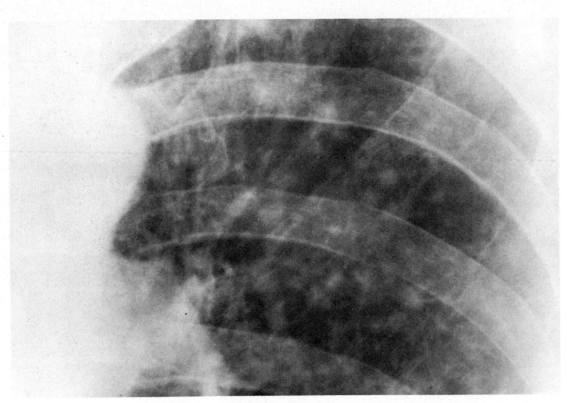

Figure B–3 Close-up

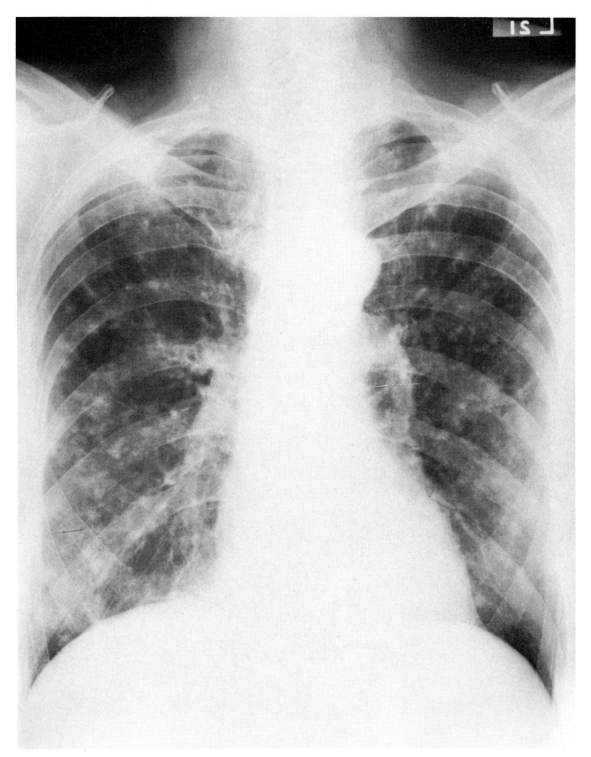

Figure B–3

Case B–3.   This patient was a 77 year old white male who presented for routine follow-up examination 14 months after colonic surgery. Do you think the radiograph demonstrates metastatic nodules?

DISCUSSION, CASE B–3

If you believe that the multiple nodules are secondary to metastatic carcinoma, you are correct. Close observation reveals that the nodules are well circumscribed, vary considerably in size, and are perfectly compatible with metastases. Although this patient may fit best in Section A, as he had surgery 14 months earlier for carcinoma of the colon, occasionally a patient will present with multiple metastatic pulmonary nodules without a known primary carcinoma. Very small, diffuse pulmonary metastatic nodules are not limited to specific primary neoplasms.

CASE B–4 _____

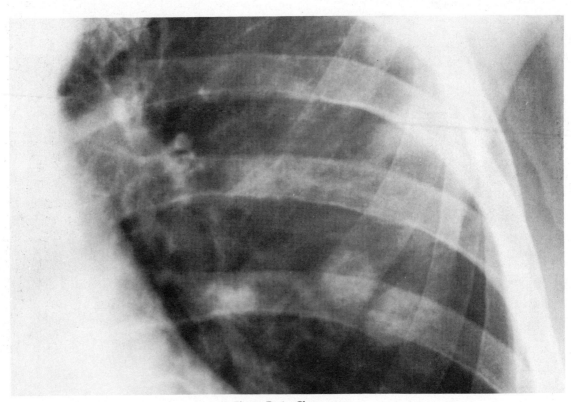

Figure B–4   Close-up

Figure B–4

Case B–4. This patient was a 41 year old white male who at the time of this radiograph had chills, fever, and a cough. Approximately 1 month before this admission he suffered a hip fracture and thereafter attempted suicide with Doriden. He survived the suicide attempt without sequelae except for a significant bone marrow depression that included the white cell series. He was admitted to the hospital with a severe urinary tract infection. What is the nature of his chest disease?

DISCUSSION, CASE B–4

This is a relatively easy case, as the historical information and the radiograph point directly toward septic emboli. On the same day the radiograph was made, a blood culture was positive for *Pseudomonas aeruginosa*. There are multiple nodules in both lungs, some of which are cavitated, and a pneumonitis is present in the right base with a small effusion. This condition is the result of embolization of septic material and is not caused by a pulmonary infarction that has become infected, which is an entirely different entity.

CASE B–5

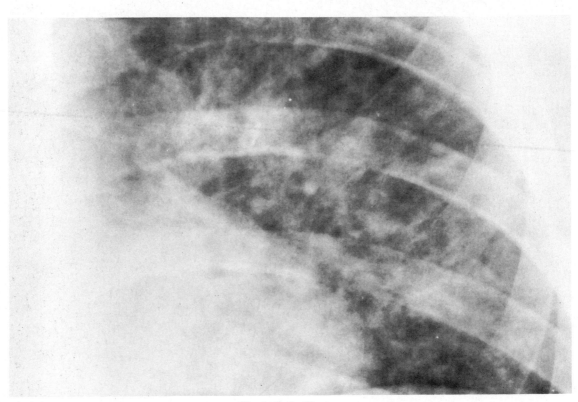

Figure B–5   Close-up

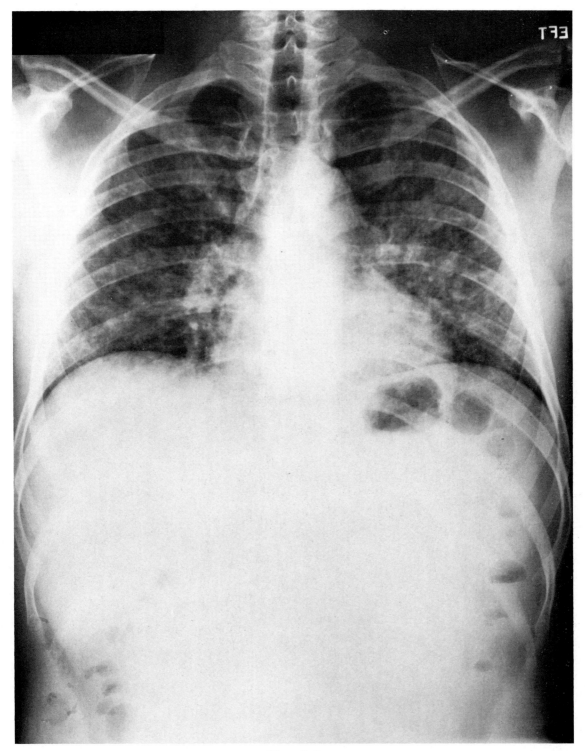

Figure B–5

Case B–5. This 40 year old white male was admitted to the hospital acutely ill with fever, cough, and dyspnea. What kind of nodules does this patient have?

DISCUSSION, CASE B–5

The patient has a multinodular disease, but the nodules do not have borders that are sharp enough to suggest metastases, and in any case, the patient is acutely ill. Airway spread of tuberculosis (not miliary) might be considered, but, although far-advanced tuberculosis may be diffuse, it is most often patchy in appearance, not nodular. In miliary tuberculosis the nodules are very much smaller and much more definitive. In this case the acute symptomatology is the key to the diagnosis, which is varicella pneumonia. Adults who develop this infection either have not been exposed as children or for some reason have no immunity. Exposure to a patient with herpes zoster or to a child with chicken pox can lead to this diffuse infection. As the lesions of varicella pneumonia heal they may calcify.

CASE B–6

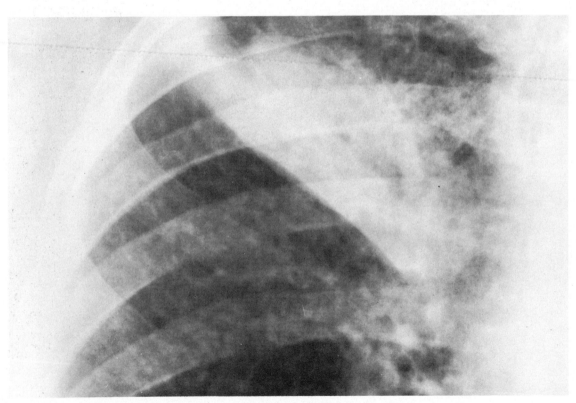

Figure B–6 Close-up

Figure B–6

Case B–6. This patient was a 62 year old white male who presented with an increasingly productive cough, weight loss, and fatigue. What kind of disease do you think this patient had? Are the nodules granulomatous, neoplastic, or caused by another process?

DISCUSSION, CASE B–6

The initial decision must determine whether the multiple small nodules are granulomatous. Then, by the proper process of elimination, one should be able to arrive at the right diagnosis. Of the common granulomatous diseases, sarcoidosis and silicosis can be virtually eliminated by this patient's age and lack of an industrial history. However, miliary tuberculosis and histoplasmosis must be kept in mind. As the multiple nodules are very much the same in size, and the margins of each are not sharply outlined, hematogenous spread of malignancy is not a likely diagnosis. The large number and the small size of the nodules as well as the absence of lymphadenopathy eliminate lymphoma as a possible diagnosis. Going on to the uncommon granulomatous diseases, we see that the lesions are far too small for us to consider rheumatoid nodules or Wegener's granulomatosis and that the patient's age and lack of industrial exposure again eliminate histiocytosis X and berylliosis. The absence of acute symptomatology or a known infection elsewhere allows us to disregard viral pneumonia or septic emboli.

Of all the possible diagnoses in Section B then, we are left with three possibilities, miliary tuberculosis, histoplasmosis, and alveolar cell carcinoma. The first two diseases must be considered, but one must account for the process in the right upper lobe, a process which is different in appearance from that of the multiple small nodules. If you now disregard the multiple small nodules and examine the right upper lobe closely, you will find that there is some loss in volume and good evidence of a primary neoplastic mass. Initial sputum smears of this patient demonstrated several acid-fast bacilli, and therefore a presumptive diagnosis of miliary tuberculosis was made. Although under the circumstances it is not incorrect to assume as a working diagnosis that the patient has miliary tuberculosis, the presence of the ominous mass makes alveolar cell carcinoma a much more likely possibility and therefore the correct choice.

CASE B–7

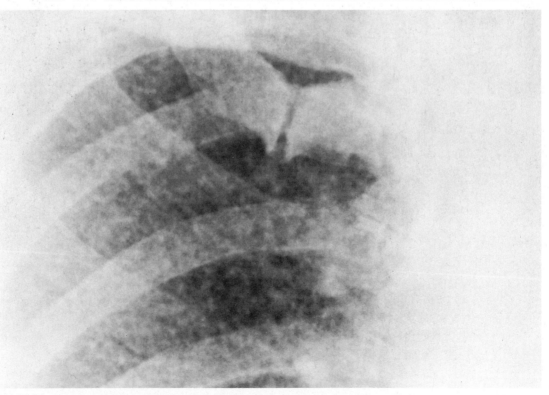

Figure B–7 Close-up

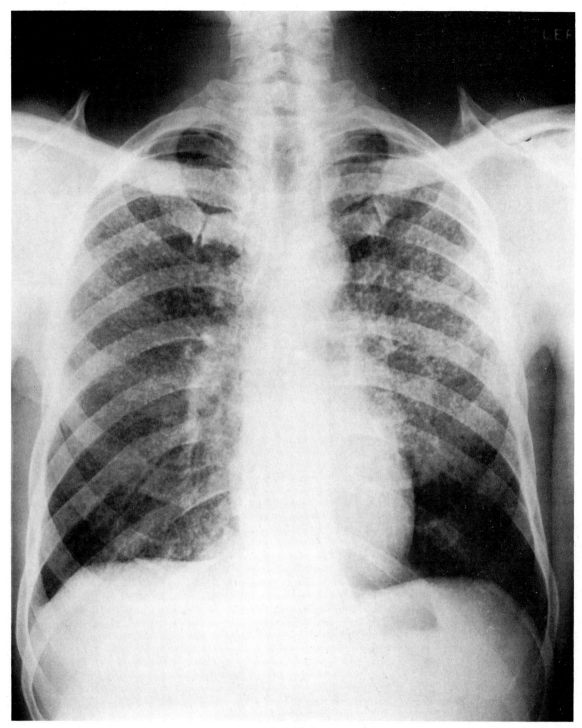

Figure B-7

Case B-7. This patient was a 32 year old male who presented with fatigue, weight loss, cough, fever, and a scrotal mass. What is your diagnosis? Are the nodules granulomatous, neoplastic, or due to another process?

DISCUSSION, CASE B–7

The nature of the scrotal mass was not clear on admission, and a testicular neoplasm could not be excluded by palpation. The radiologic diagnosis, however, should be clear, and if your diagnosis is metastases from a testicular neoplasm, you are dead wrong. The patient clearly has miliary tuberculosis as well as tuberculous epididymitis. Look at the nodules. They are very small, practically the same in size except for radiologic conglomeration, and rather evenly spread throughout both lungs. In this case, however, there is no evidence of reinfection tuberculosis. Although you might want to consider other granulomatous diseases, the appearance of the chest radiograph makes the diagnosis of miliary tuberculosis the primary one. Errors in diagnosis are made all the time, but if you can choose your error, choose the one that is safe for the patient. It is better to be wrong in diagnosing miliary tuberculosis than wrong in not diagnosing it.

CASE B–8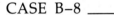

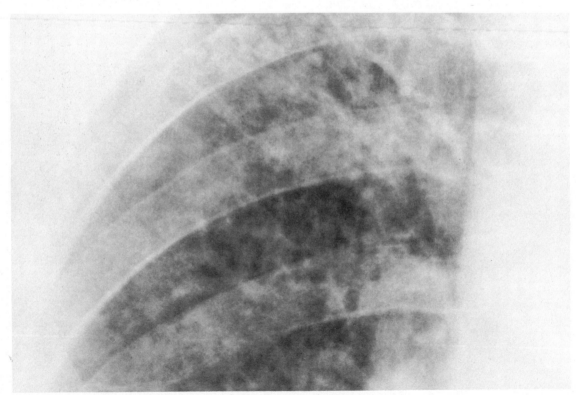

Figure B–8   Close-up

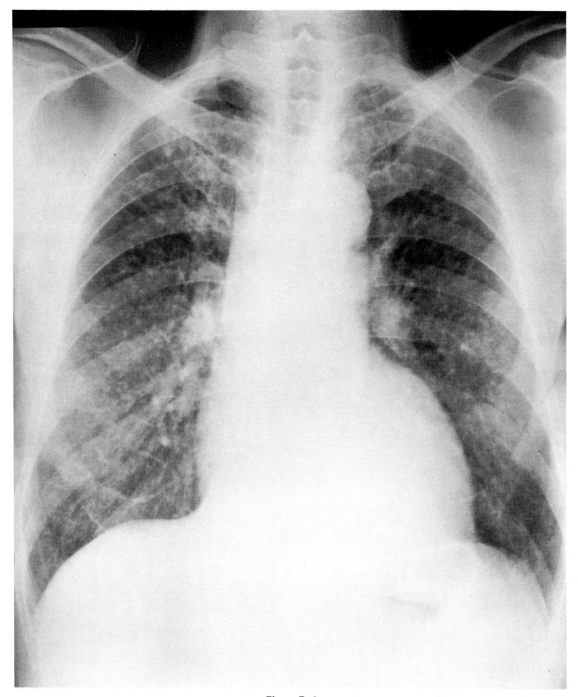

Figure B–8

Case B–8.   This patient was a 67 year old white male who complained of increasing dyspnea when he presented for a routine follow-up examination. What would be your first choice of diagnoses? Are the nodules granulomatous or neoplastic?

DISCUSSION, CASE B–8

This patient was a hard coal miner and undoubtedly had coal worker's pneumoconiosis but may have had silicosis as well. The role that free silica plays in the development of coal worker's pneumoconiosis is still controversial, but it is most likely that carbon dust itself can cause the disease. In this text, however, silicosis and pneumoconiosis will be considered together.

In making the first decision we note that the nodules are approximately the same in size, the margins of each nodule are irregular and that the nodules are found predominantly in the upper lobes. Some patients with silicosis have calcified lymphadenopathy in the hila, but many do not. In addition, there may be considerable superimposed fibrosis and compensatory hyperaeration, which make the diagnosis even easier.

In this case the patient's increasing dyspnea was probably due to early heart failure, as his heart is enlarged, although he does not show signs of failure in his lungs.

CASE B–9 _____

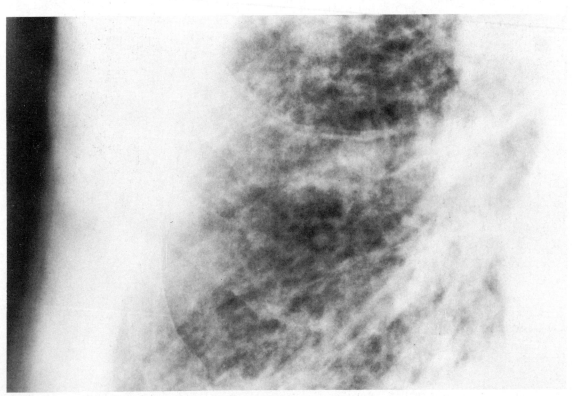

Figure B–9a   Close-up

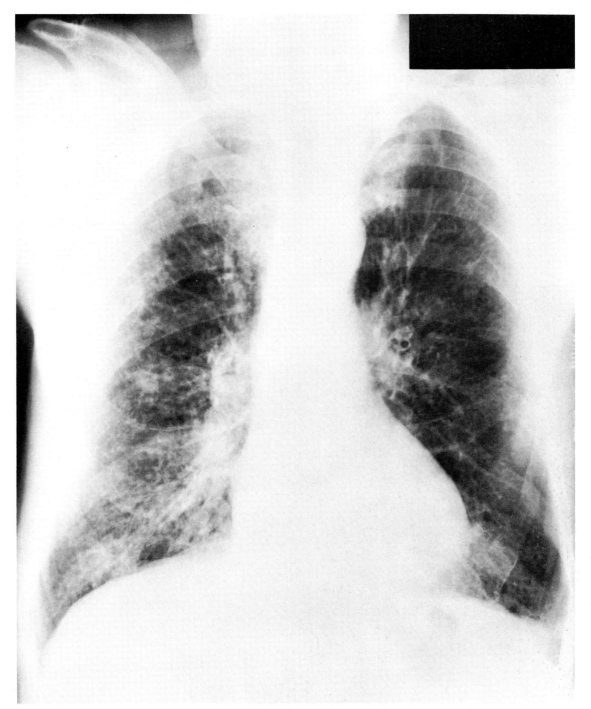

Figure B–9a

Case B–9. This patient was a 61 year old white male who presented with acute dyspnea. For many years he had had a productive chronic cough and moderate dyspnea on exertion. Why do you think this patient has acute dyspnea at this time? What type of nodular disease do you think is present?

A radiograph made following therapy is on the next page, but try to make your diagnosis before turning to it.

CASE B-9 *CONTINUED*

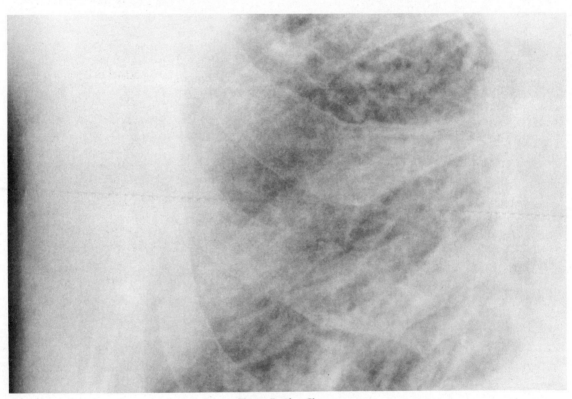

Figure B-9b   Close-up

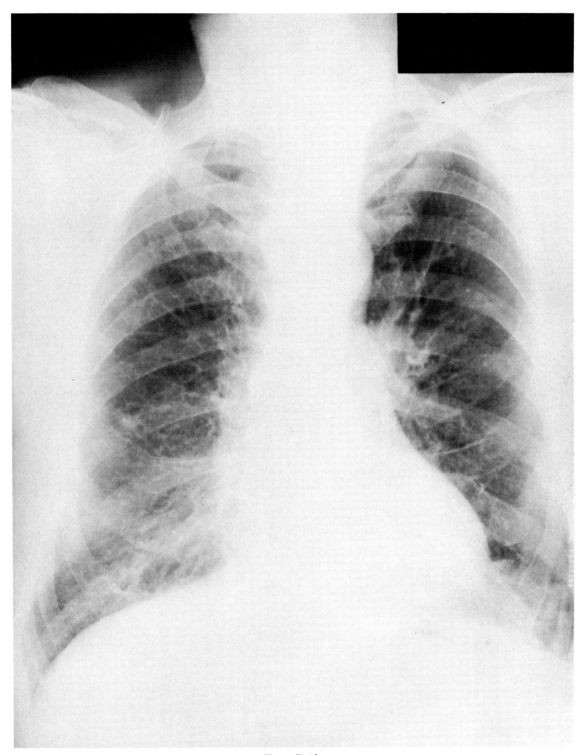

Figure B-9b

Case B-9b. This is the same patient as demonstrated in Figure B-9a, 1 week later. After appropriate therapy the pulmonary edema has cleared, although the heart remains larger than expected in a hyperaerated chest.

DISCUSSION, CASE B–9

If your diagnosis is congestive heart failure superimposed on chronic obstructive airways disease, you are absolutely correct. The recognition of heart failure in a patient with obstructive airways disease may be very difficult, but it is also crucial. One of the more unusual presentations of heart failure is the nodular form of pulmonary edema, which is dependent upon the nature of the underlying chronic lung disease. It should be observed that this patient has a nodular pattern in the right lower lobe only, and this is one clue to the diagnosis. He is demonstrating heart failure only where he has a sufficient remaining pulmonary vascular bed.

The problem in this case is not so much to differentiate between granulomata and metastases — as is often the case when a patient presents with multiple nodules — as it is to recognize an unusual pattern of pulmonary edema. This subject will be discussed more fully in Section C.

CASE B–10

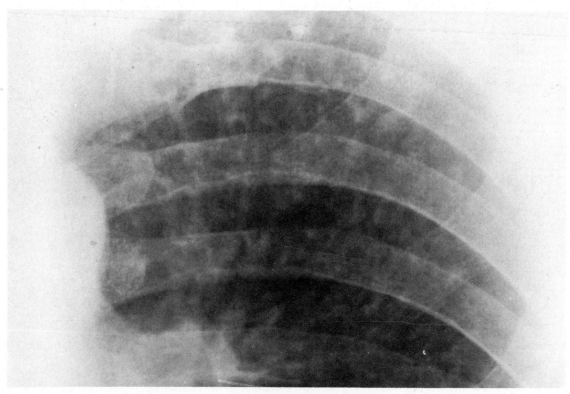

Figure B–10   Close-up

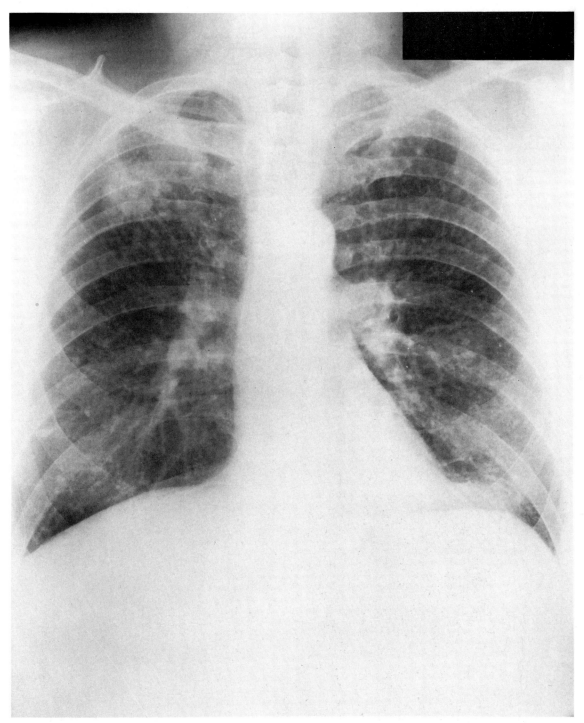

Figure B–10

Case B–10. This patient was a 57 year old white male who presented with a chronic cough. Are the nodules granulomatous, neoplastic, or due to another process? What is the nature of the larger nodule on the right side?

DISCUSSION, CASE B–10

This is another case of coal worker's pneumoconiosis, once again in a miner of anthracite coal. The essential question in this case, after the diagnosis of pneumoconiosis or silicosis is made, however, revolves around the cause of the lesion in the right upper lobe. There are three possibilities — a conglomerate mass secondary to the patient's silicosis, tuberculosis, or primary carcinoma of the lung. Which do you favor? Never trust a unilateral conglomerate mass, even if the patient has known silicosis and particularly if there is no other suggestion of conglomeration on either side. Further evaluation at the time of presentation was definitely indicated in this case. A primary neoplasm could not be excluded as a diagnosis, but several months later the lesion underwent cavitation, and the presence of active tuberculosis was proved.

CASE B–11

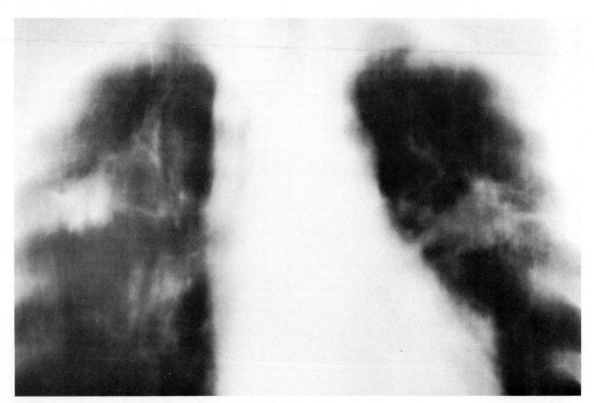

Figure B–11   Close-up

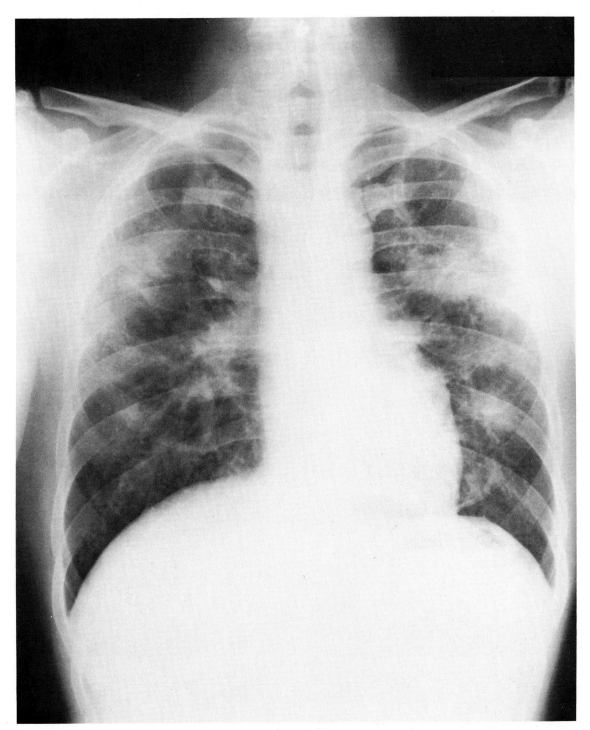

Figure B–11

Case B–11. This patient was a 44 year old white male who presented with hypertension, headaches, polyuria, and proteinuria. (The close-up is a photograph of a tomogram of the upper lobes.) Can you put this case together? Are the lesions granulomatous, neoplastic, or caused by another disease?

DISCUSSION, CASE B–11

This patient has multiple, grossly irregular pulmonary lesions, at least one of which is cavitated. The absence of mutliple small nodules eliminates most of the common granulomatous diseases, but two granulomatous processes merit consideration. In a silicotic patient it is quite unlikely, but possible, for all the nodules to be drawn into conglomerate masses. The absence of an industrial history in this patient, however, eliminates this possibility. Of the infections that cause granulomata, only nocardiosis should be considered with this roentgen appearance. Because the lesions are not sharply outlined, a metastatic neoplasm is a highly unlikely possibility. Rheumatoid nodules are usually smoother in outline than these lesions, and the patient most often has evidence of rheumatoid arthritis, which is not present in this patient. Wegener's granulomatosis, however, is not only entirely possible but is the best diagnostic possibility in this case, particularly in light of the evidence of a process involving multiple organ systems.

CASE B–12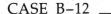

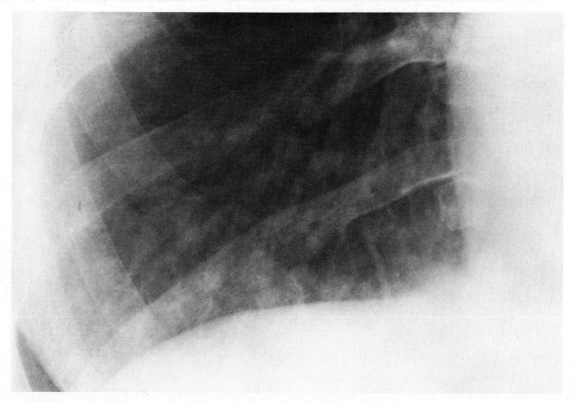

Figure B–12   Close-up

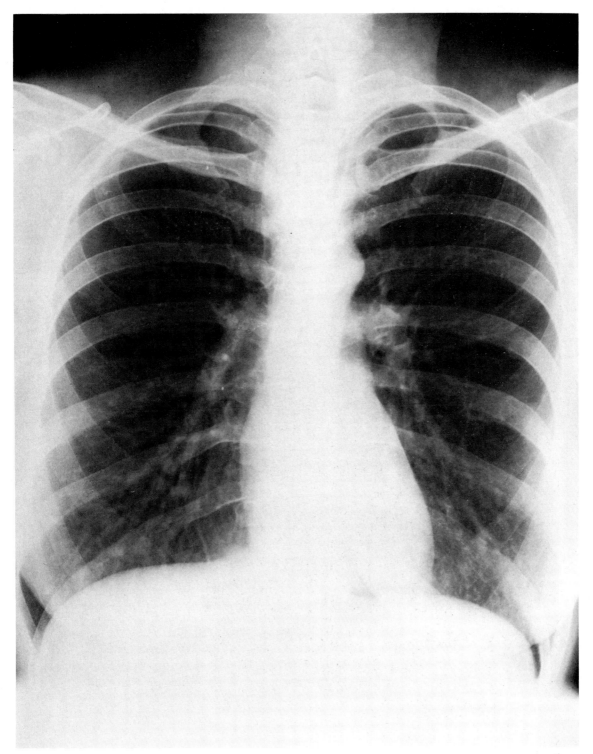

Figure B–12

Case B–12. This patient was a 45 year old asymptomatic hospital volunteer who presented for a routine annual chest examination. You should be able to make this diagnosis.

DISCUSSION, CASE B–12

The multiple nodules are well defined, variable in size, and in the lower lobes. If these clues do not give you the diagnosis in this asymptomatic individual, then noting the superior mediastinal mass that deviates the trachea toward the left certainly should. The correct diagnosis is metastatic colloid-producing carcinoma of the thyroid. The patient underwent surgery, and the superior mediastinal mass was found to be a carcinoma. The metastatic nodules were cleared by therapy with radioactive iodine.

CASE B–13 _____

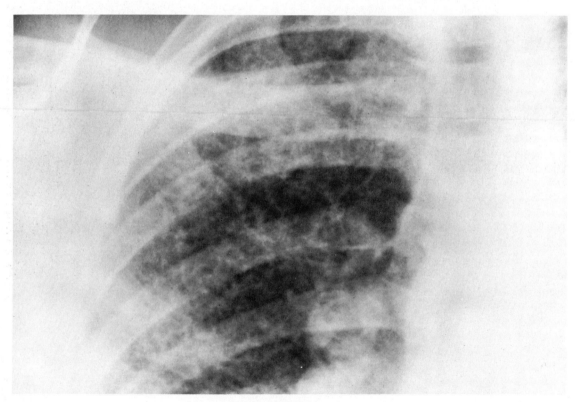

Figure B–13   Close-up

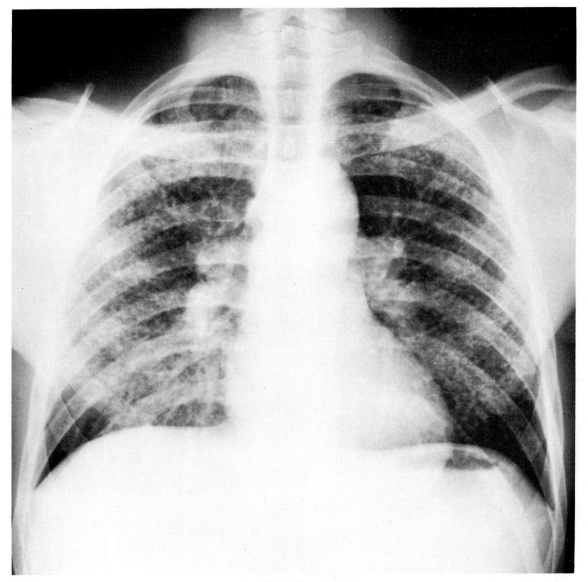

Figure B-13

Case B-13. This patient was a 21 year old black male who presented with increasing dyspnea and a dry cough. Look carefully; there are nodules present, but are they granulomatous, neoplastic, or neither? What is your differential diagnosis?

DISCUSSION, CASE B–13

Close observation reveals multiple, very small nodules, which are approximately the same size and irregular in outline. This and the history certainly put the nodules into the granulomatous category. Further observation reveals a cystic component of this diffuse parenchymal disease. You are right if you think that miliary tuberculosis must be ruled out. Although it is not the correct diagnosis, it certainly cannot be entirely eliminated on the basis of the radiographic appearance and clinical history alone. Sarcoidosis, even without lymphadenopathy, histiocytosis X, and histoplasmosis must also be considered. An industrial disease would not be likely in this 21 year old patient and can be eliminated on the basis of the absence of exposure indicated by history. The patient was not acutely ill and has no evidence of other organ system involvement. The diagnois in this young black male, considering all the conceivable parameters prior to biopsy, is either histiocytosis X or sarcoidosis. In this case, sarcoidosis can be eliminated only by biopsy. However, the diffuse nature of the process, which is somewhat more marked in the upper lobes, the presence of a moderate fibrotic component, the small granulomata, and the cysts make a diagnosis of histiocytosis X the most likely possibility. In this case the results of the biopsy were consistent with the diagnosis of eosinophilic granuloma.

A more undifferentiated form of the disease, usually called malignant histiocytosis or histiocytic medullary reticulosis, is also found, but it is quite rare. There is probably a spectrum of histiocytic disorders ranging from the most differentiated eosinophilic granuloma to the least differentiated diffuse histiocytic lymphoma. Malignant histiocytosis occupies a middle position on this spectrum.

CASE B–14

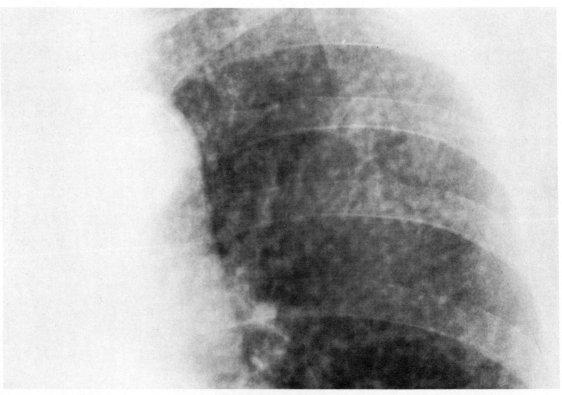

Figure B–14   Close-up

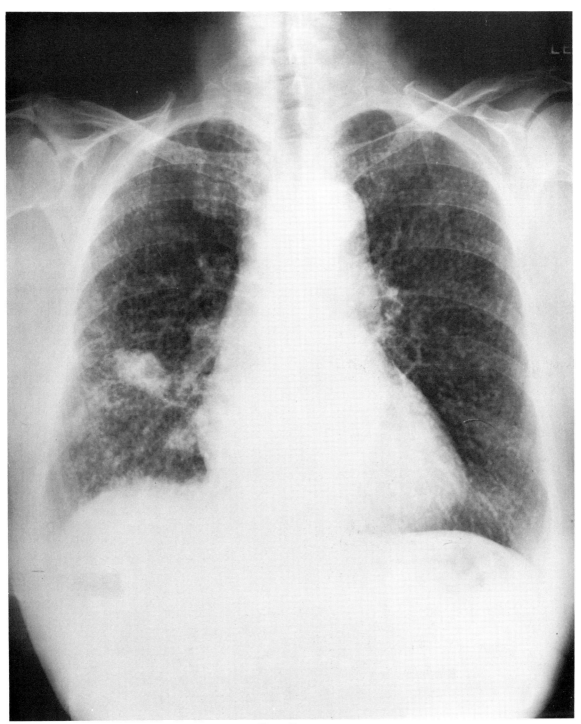

Figure B–14

Case B–14. This patient was a 72 year old white female who presented with increasing dyspnea and a productive cough during the several weeks prior to admission. There was no industrial history. Are the nodules granulomatous, neoplastic, or caused by some other entity? What is your differential diagnosis?

DISCUSSION, CASE B–14

This case should now be relatively straightforward, as the similarity to the earlier case of alveolar cell carcinoma is striking. There are multiple small nodules that represent clumps of acini filled with neoplasm. The primary mass is not as striking as in the earlier case, but it is certainly obvious in the right lower chest. A well-circumscribed tuberculoma or histoplasmoma is not expected in the same chest with widespread miliary tuberculosis or histoplasmosis.

Alveolar cell carcinoma presents most often as a solitary small mass, but in a significant percentage of the cases multiple tiny nodules are present as well as a mass of some type. These multiple tiny nodules are acini filled with carcinoma, not hematogenously distributed nodules in the interstitium. (Alveolar cell carcinoma has other, even more bizarre presentations that resemble solitary or multiple areas of pulmonary consolidation.)

CASE B–15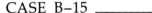

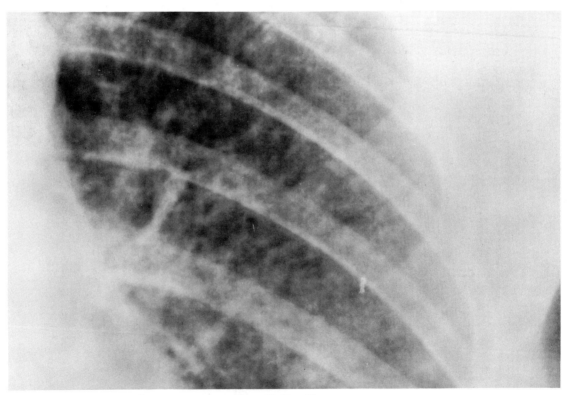

Figure B–15a   Close-up

Figure B–15a

Case B–15a. This patient was a 32 year old black female who presented with dyspnea and a chronic cough for the past 4 weeks. She had been entirely well previously. What is your diagnosis? A later radiograph follows.

DISCUSSION, CASE B–15

Once again we are dealing with multiple small nodules that are irregular in outline but approximately the same in size. The disease is somewhat more marked in the central portion of the right lung but is otherwise quite diffuse. Although the lesions are larger than expected with miliary tuberculosis, this disease must be considered, along with sarcoidosis and possibly histiocytosis X. The correct diagnosis in this case is sarcoidosis. There is a certain linearity to some of the areas, but no true fibrosis can be seen. It is, however, difficult to ascertain exactly when the complications of sarcoidosis, most commonly fibrosis and cyst formation, appear. The presence of lymphadenopathy is questionable in this case. The patient's age and race help in establishing the radiographic diagnosis.

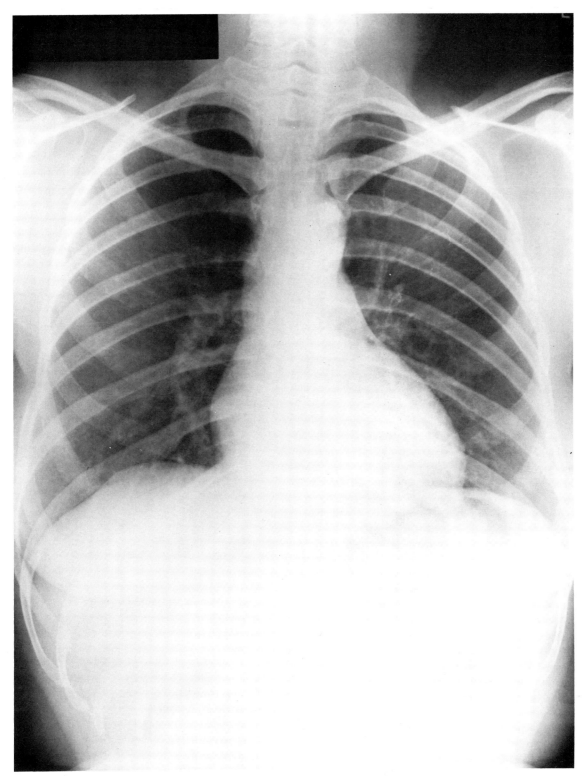

Figure B–15b

Case B–15b. This is a radiograph of the same patient shown in Figure B–15a almost 2 years later. There is no evidence of residual parenchymal disease at this time, and in retrospect right azygous lymphadenopathy was probably evident in the earlier radiograph.

CASE B–16 _____

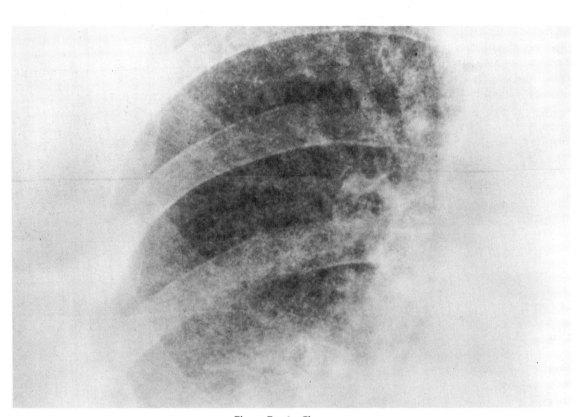

Figure B–16   Close-up

Figure B–16

Case B–16. This patient was an asymptomatic 46 year old white female. The radiograph on this page and those on the five succeeding pages all illustrate diffuse pulmonary calcifications. While identification of the exact nature of the pulmonary calcification is usually of little clinical importance in the individual patient, it helps us as radiologists to understand the natural history of various disease processes. Clearly, it is more of a diagnostic game than anything else, but why not see how well you can do? One clue—the etiology of the calcifications is different in each of the six patients. Discussion of these cases in on page 99.

CASE B–17 _____

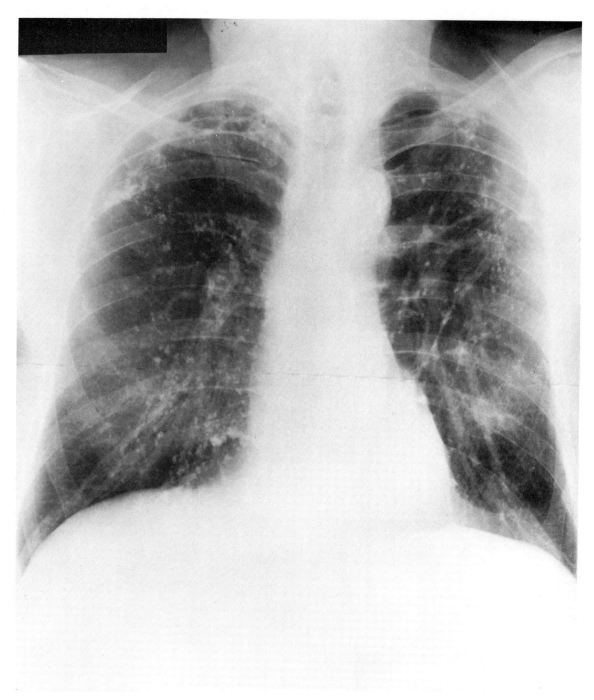

Figure B–17

Case B–17.   This patient was an asymptomatic 58 year old white male.

CASE B–18

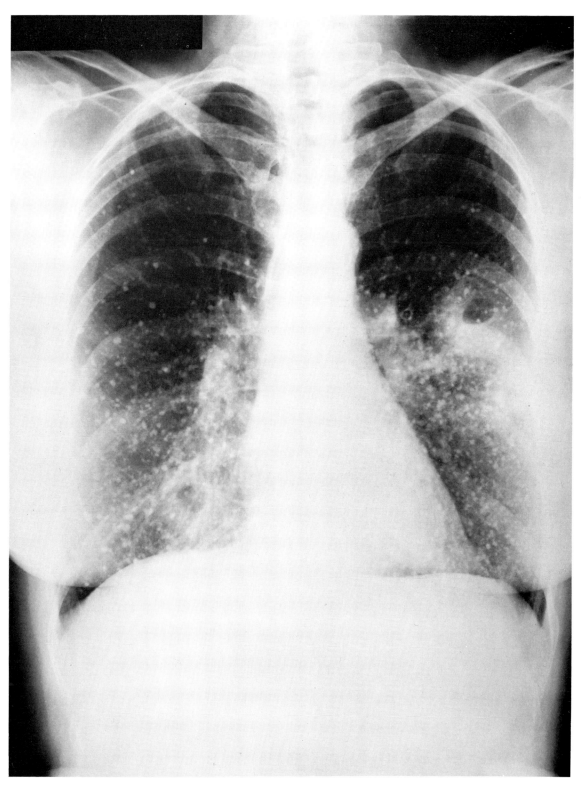

Figure B–18

Case B–18.   The patient was a 54 year old white female who presented with septic thrombophlebitis of the left leg. The calcifications and the cavitated lesions are not caused by the same process.

CASE B–19 _____

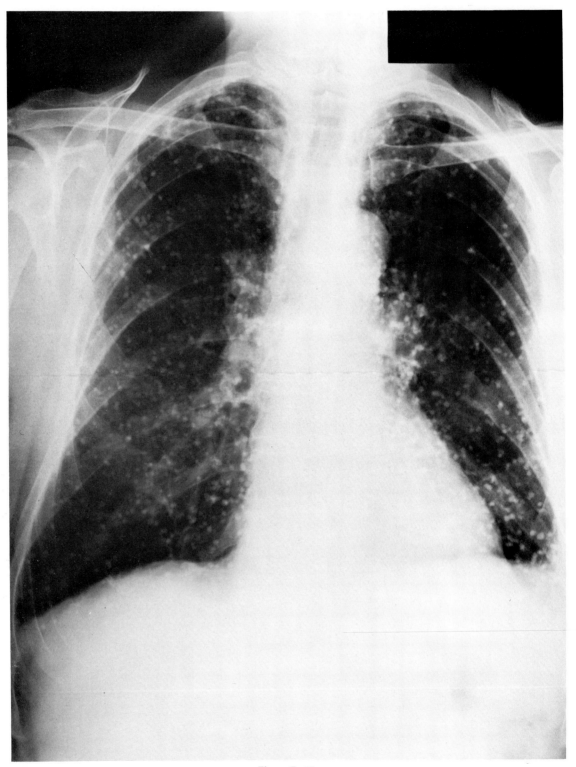

Figure B–19

Case B–19.   This patient was an asymptomatic 42 year old white male.

CASE B–20 _____

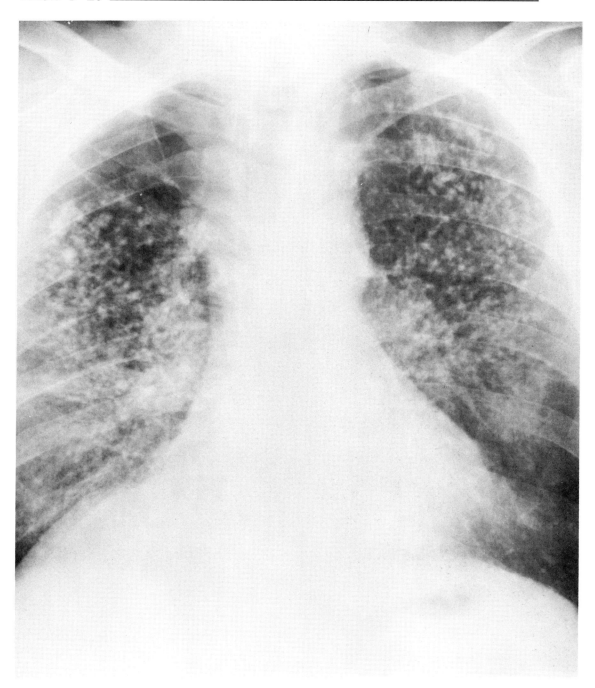

Figure B–20

Case B–20. This patient was a 69 year old white male who presented with moderate dyspnea on exertion and a chronic cough.

CASE B–21 _____

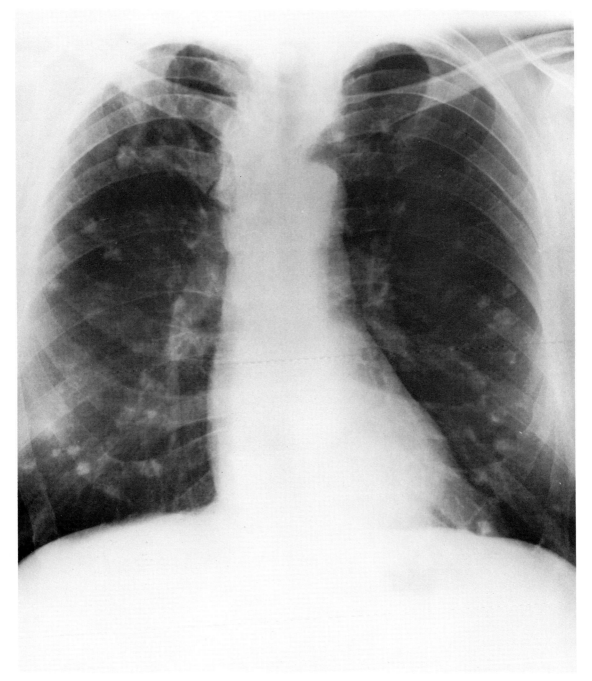

Figure B–21

Case B–21. This patient was an asymptomatic 54 year old white male.

DISCUSSION, CASES B–16 through B–21

Case B–16, Pulmonary Alveolar Micro-lithiasis

The recognition of this entity, the etiology of which is unknown, is not difficult. The calcifications are finely granular because they are in the alveolar spaces; no other disease presents with quite the same radiographic appearance. The patients are almost always asymptomatic, and occasionally the lungs become so dense that the pleura is seen as a radiolucent stripe between the calcifications in the pulmonary parenchyma and the rib cage.

Case B–17,   Tuberculosis

Diffuse pulmonary tuberculous calcifications can be recognized by the clumped appearance of the calcific lesions as well as by the associated fibrosis. The calcifications of tuberculosis are not evenly distributed, as miliary tuberculosis does not calcify, and airway spread is most often well localized. One should also note that the individual calcified lesions are grossly irregular and quite variable in size and shape.

Case B–18, Calcified Varicella Pneumonia (and unrelated septic emboli)

The calcifications of varicella pneumonia are rare, but a significant group of patients with this disease was reported from Australia some years ago. The appearance of the calcifications is quite different from that in the two preceding cases, as in this case lesions are in the interstitium of the lung, not in the alveolar spaces, and they are not as clumped and grossly irregular as those secondary to tuberculosis.

Case B–19, Histoplasmosis

The calcifications of histoplasmosis are the easiest of any to recognize, as the lesions appear smooth in outline when contrasted with the lesions of other diseases that cause pulmonary calcifications. They are fairly widely and evenly distributed throughout the lungs, and are regular in size. Calcification of hilar lymph nodes may be seen as well. Calcified diffuse histoplasmosis is probably the most common of all diffuse pulmonary calcifications.

Case B-20, Calcific Pulmonary Silicosis

This patient was a copper miner, and like coal workers, copper miners suffered from industrial pneumoconiosis prior to the introduction of modern safety measures. Calcification of the nodules to the degree seen in this case, however, is uncommon. The entity may be recognized by the upper lobe distribution that is expected in silicotics as well as by the evidence of lymphadenopathy, some of which is calcified.

Case B–21, Coccidioidomycosis

These calcified lesions are an exceedingly rare manifestion of a disease common in the southwestern United States. The individual lesions are much larger than those expected in histoplasmosis or varicella pneumonia. The distribution of the lesions rules against silicosis, as does the absence of secondary fibrosis and lymphadenopathy. It is conceivable that tuberculosis as well as other fungal infections could cause calcifications of this nature.

REFERENCES

1. Berkmen, Y.: The many faces of bronchioalveolar cell carcinoma. Semin. Roentgenol., 12:207–214, 1977.
2. Dunnick, N. R., Parker, B. R., Warnke, R. A., et al.: Radiographic manifestations of malignant histiocytosis. Am. J. Roentgenol., 127:611–616, 1976.
3. Freundlich, I. M., Libshitz, H. I., Glassman, L. M., et al.: Sarcoidosis. Typical and atypical thoracic manifestations and complications. Clin. Radiol., 21:376–383, 1970.
4. Gilsanz, V., and Harris, G. B. C.: Histiocytic medullary reticulosis in childhood. Radiology, 126:463–465, 1978.
5. Hublitz, U. F., and Shapiro, J. H.: Atypical pulmonary patterns of congestive failure in chronic lung disease. Radiology, 93:995–1006, 1969.
6. Jones, R. N., and Weill, H.: Occupational lung disease. Basics of RD, Vol. 6, No. 3, pp. 1–6. American Thoracic Society, 1978.
7. Kirks, D. R., and Greenspan, R. H.: Sarcoid. Radiol. Clin. North Am., 11(2):279–294, 1973.
8. Knyvett, A., Stringer, R., and Abrahams, E.: The radiology of chicken-pox lung. J. Coll. Radiol. Aust., 9:134–139, 1965.
9. Ludington, L. G., Verska, J. J., Howard, T., et al.: Bronchiolar carcinoma (alveolar cell), another great imitator; a review of 41 cases. Chest, 61(7):622–628, 1972.
10. Morgan, W. K. C., and Lapp, L.: Respiratory disease in coal miners. In Murray, J. F. (ed.): Lung Disease — State of the Art 1975–1976. New York, American Lung Association, 1977, pp. 28–29.
11. Pump, K. K.: Studies in silicosis of the human lung. Dis. Chest, 53(3):237–246, 1968.
12. Rabinowitz, J. G., Busch, J., and Buttram, W. R.: Pulmonary manifestations of blastomycosis. Radiology, 120:25–32, 1976.
13. Ziskind, M., Jones, R. N., and Weill, H.: Silicosis. In Murray, J. F. (ed.): Lung Disease — State of the Art 1975–1976. New York, American Lung Association, 1977, pp. 1–23.

If the answers to the questions posed in Sections A and B are no, that is, the patient is not immunosuppressed and the roentgenographic appearance of the diffuse pulmonary disease is not nodular, then we are ready to ask the third question. Is the disease predominantly an *airspace filling process?*

Decision 1. If the disease is an airspace filling process, then Decision 1 is obvious — does the patient have pulmonary edema? While pulmonary edema may be central and symmetric in its distribution, hydrostatic edema is gravity-dependent, and therefore the patient's body position will play a role in its distribution. Pulmonary edema that is related to injury to the capillary endothelium and to an increase in the permeability of the alveolocapillary membrane will tend to have a fixed distribution, in contrast to purely hydrostatic edema.

Although by common usage the escape of intravascular fluid and possibly other blood products into the lung is called "pulmonary edema," the mechanism of injury to the alveolocapillary membrane suggests that a number of these entities should probably be termed "pneumonitis."

Some of the more common causes of pulmonary edema are listed as follows, and clearly history is essential:

A. hydrostatic pulmonary edema
   1. cardiac failure
   2. overhydration (generalized venous congestion with no redistribution)
   3. heroin overdose
B. injury to the alveolocapillary membrane

   1. renal failure
   2. shock
      a. septic shock
      b. neurogenic shock
   3. inhalation of toxic substances
   4. near drowning

(*Note:* Interstitial pulmonary edema may precede airspace edema in any of the entities just listed.)

Decision 2. Does the patient have congestive heart failure or is he overhydrated? Although acute pulmonary edema often will not demonstrate the signs of chronic congestive heart failure, the radiologist should look for the following signs:

   a. increased heart size
   b. venous congestion
   c. venous redistribution
   d. edematous interstitial septa (Kerley's lines)
   e. pleural and subpleural effusions

Decision 3. Decision 3 involves the possibility of congestive heart failure superimposed upon chronic obstructive pulmonary disease. Unusual patterns of pulmonary edema may be seen in the acutely dyspneic patients who have this disorder, and close examination of any available earlier radiographs is mandatory. Hublitz and Shapiro[6] have described four patterns seen in these patients:

   a. regional
   b. interstitial
   c. reticular
   d. miliary-nodular

Decision 4. Decision 4 is made on the basis of evidence in the patient's his-

101

tory of inhalation of toxic substances, near drowning, heroin overdose, uremia, or any other cause of pulmonary edema. In cases with such a history, the pulmonary edema may be distributed in an unusual fashion, with patches of edema scattered diffusely throughout the lungs. Uremic pulmonary edema (uremic pneumonitis) probably fits best in this category, although it is most frequently central and symmetric in its distribution. Cardiac and renal pulmonary edema may often be present simultaneously.

Pulmonary edema is rarely encountered unexpectedly, and a significant concomitant history should always be available. This is occasionally not the case with patients suffering from the chronic inhalation of noxious gases.

Decision 5.   Decision 5 is the consideration of those hospital patients who might have the adult respiratory distress syndrome (ARDS). The development of this entity, which has also been called respiratory lung, shock lung, and bronchopulmonary dysplasia, is related to the extent of damage to the alveolocapillary membrane. Therefore, it is not unexpected for ARDS to develop following any severe diffuse pulmonary insult. The etiology of the underlying disease is not as important as the extent of the damage that that disease has done to the permeability of the alveolocapillary membrane. A few of the entities that lead to the adult respiratory distress syndrome are as follows:

a. oxygen toxicity
b. disseminated intravascular coagulation (DIC)

c. septic shock
d. fat embolization

Decision 6.   If a diffuse airspace filling process is present, and there is no known cause of pulmonary edema, then we move to Decision 6, the consideration of one of the following unusual entities:

a. pulmonary alveolar proteinosis
b. pulmonary hemorrhage (hemosiderosis)
1. hemorrhage secondary to mitral valvular disease
2. Goodpasture's syndrome
3. leukemia or thrombocytopenia
4. idiopathic hemosiderosis
c. eosinophilic pneumonia (type III immune response)
1. acute, transient pneumonia (Löffler's pneumonia)
2. chronic eosinophilic pneumonia

Pulmonary alveolar proteinosis is characterized by insignificant or minimal symptomatology and, in contrast, by a roentgenogram that shows a significant alveolar filling process. The discrepancy between the radiographic findings and the symptomatology is frequently the best clue to the diagnosis. Hemosiderosis, which is diagnosed most often when macrophages containing hemosiderin are found in the sputum or in a gastric aspiration, Goodpasture's syndrome, and eosinophilic pneumonia may be considered to be alveolar filling processes, but they fit best in Section E, which deals with the hypersensitivity reactions.

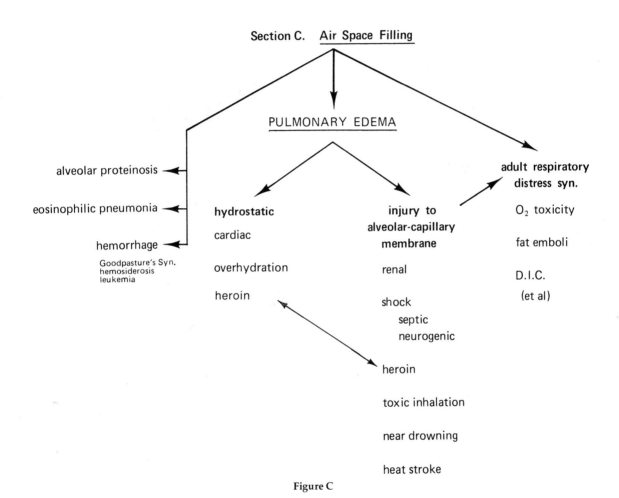

Section C.   Air Space Filling

PULMONARY EDEMA

alveolar proteinosis

eosinophilic pneumonia

hemorrhage

Goodpasture's Syn.
hemosiderosis
leukemia

hydrostatic

cardiac

overhydration

heroin

**injury to
alveolar-capillary
membrane**

renal

shock
  septic
  neurogenic

heroin

toxic inhalation

near drowning

heat stroke

**adult respiratory
distress syn.**

O_2 toxicity

fat emboli

D.I.C.

(et al)

Figure C

CASE C–1 _____

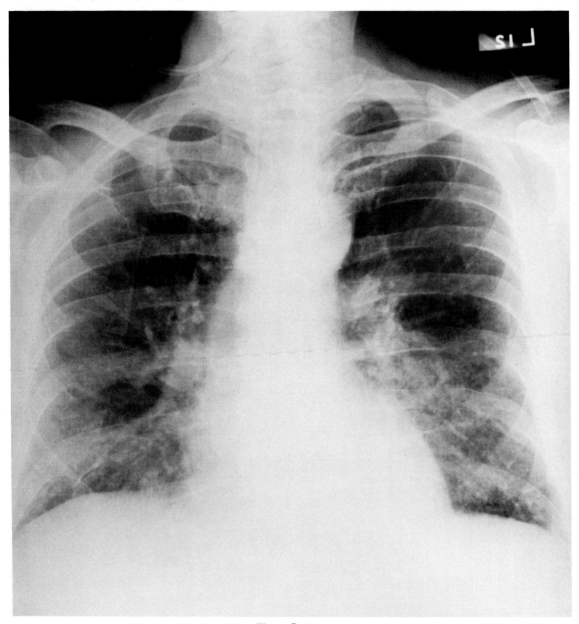

Figure C–1a

Case C–1a. This patient was a 75 year old white male who presented with acute dyspnea and abdominal pain (Fig. C–1a). The patient's past medical history is remarkable in that he had had a myocardial infarction. He had no other known illnesses. Additional radiographs of this patient are seen on the next two pages.

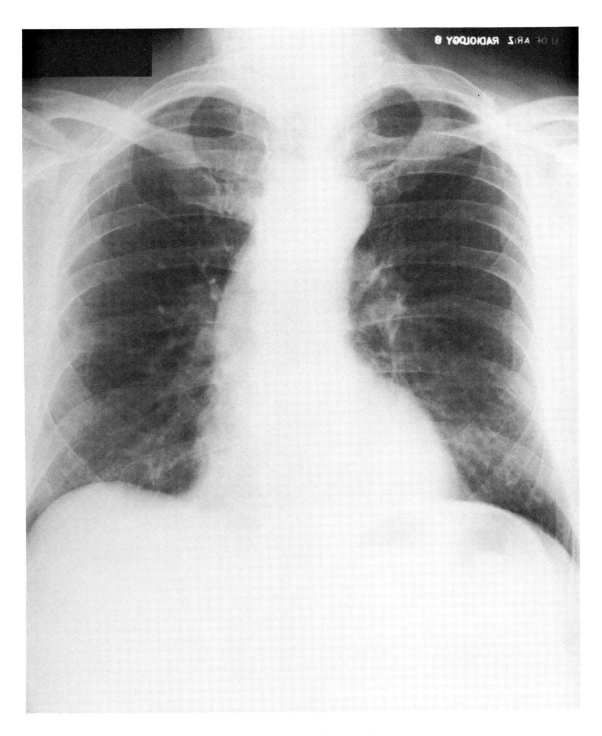

Figure C–1b

Case C –1b. This radiograph of the same patient was made 3 years before the radiograph shown in Fig. C–1a.

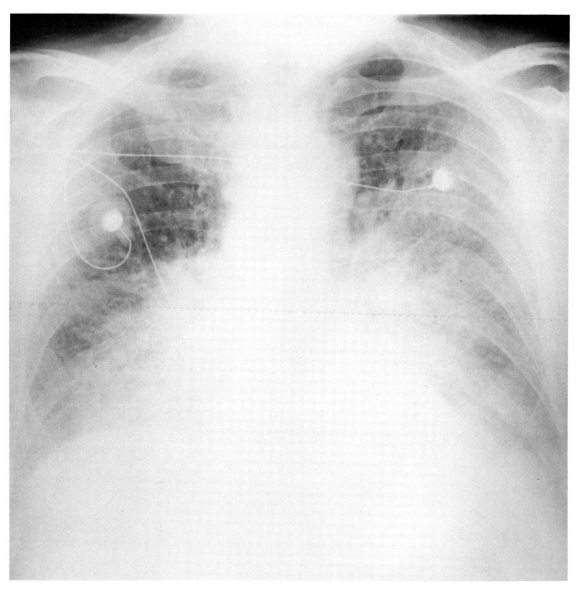

Figure C–1c

Case C–1c. This radiograph of the same patient was made approximately 24 hours after the radiograph shown in Figure C–1a.

DISCUSSION, CASE C–1

This man has a common radiographic picture of pulmonary edema. The pattern is typical in that it is mostly central and symmetric and somewhat more marked in the lower lobes.

It is, however, essential in this case that the diagnosis be made as early as possible so that the proper treatment may be rapidly initiated. On pages 104 and 105 are radiographs of the patient made approximately 3 years before this admission (Fig. C–1b) and at the time of this admission (Fig. C–1a), when the diagnosis was made. Note the interstitial pulmonary edema, which includes edematous bronchial walls, although the heart size remains within normal limits. It is not unusual for patients with acute heart failure secondary to a myocardial infarction to have hearts of a normal size. It should also be noted that the signs of chronic or slowly progressive left ventricular decompensation are *not* present. These signs include redistribution of pulmonary blood flow to the upper lobes, edematous interstitial septa (Kerley's B lines), and pleural effusion. It is just as important, if not more so, to make the diagnosis of acute heart failure when the radiograph shows only interstitial edema as when more obvious signs are present.

Hydrostatic pulmonary edema is gravity-dependent. This is not the case for those causes of pulmonary edema that are related to altered permeability of the alveolocapillary membrane. Nonhydrostatic pulmonary edema, which in most cases is probably best called pneumonitis, is not gravity-dependent, as the alveolar and interstitial transudate or exudate will be present at the site of the injury to the alveolocapillary membrane. Of course, there are cases in which the water in the lungs is caused in part by hydrostatic edema and in part by damage to the alveolocapillary membrane.

CASE C–2 _____

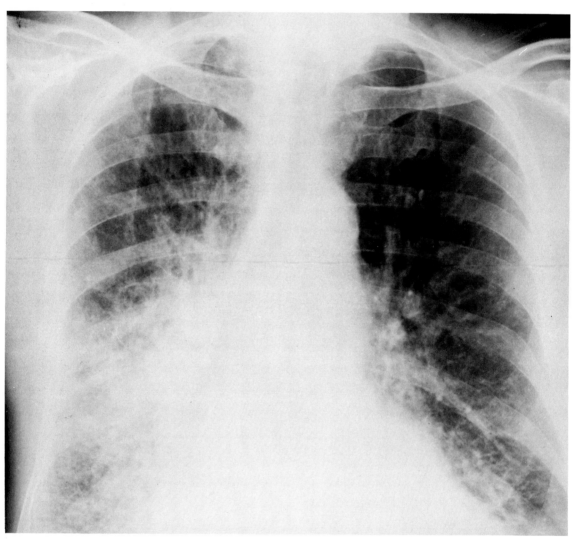

Figure C–2a

Case C–2a. This patient was a 75 year old white male who presented in congestive heart failure with predominantly right-sided pulmonary edema.

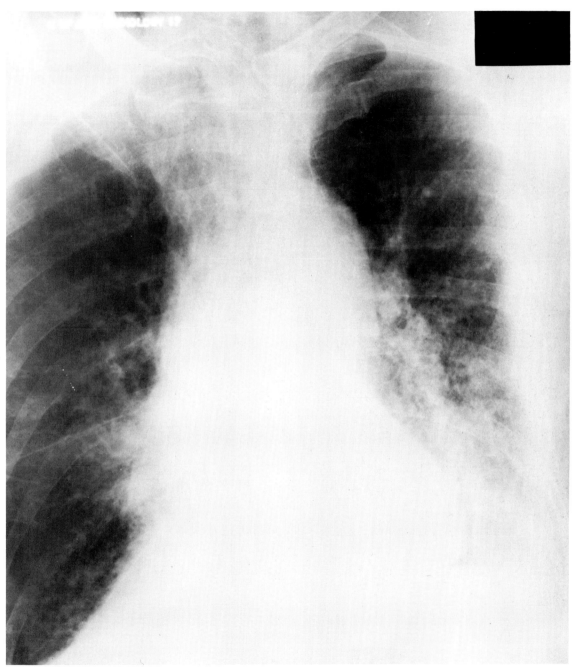

Figure C–2b

Case C–2b.   How did the pulmonary edema shift?

DISCUSSION, CASE C–2

Left lateral decubitus examination of the same patient shown in Figure C–2a less than 1 hour after the radiograph on the preceding page was made demonstrates the phenomenon of "shifting pulmonary edema" (Fig. C–2b). Actually, of course, the edema does not shift but disappears where the pressure is diminished, in this case in the right lung, and reappears in the left lung, where the pressure is increased when the patient is in the left lateral decubitus position.

CASE C–3

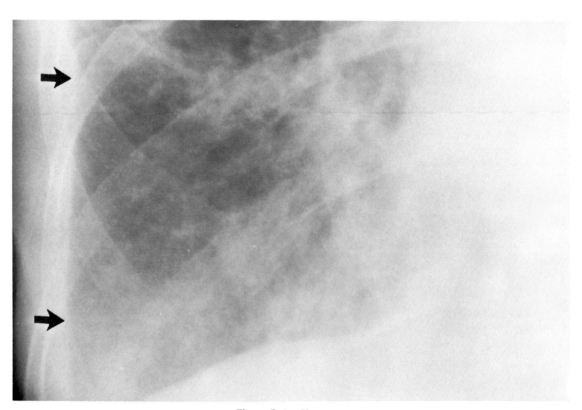

Figure C–3   Close-up

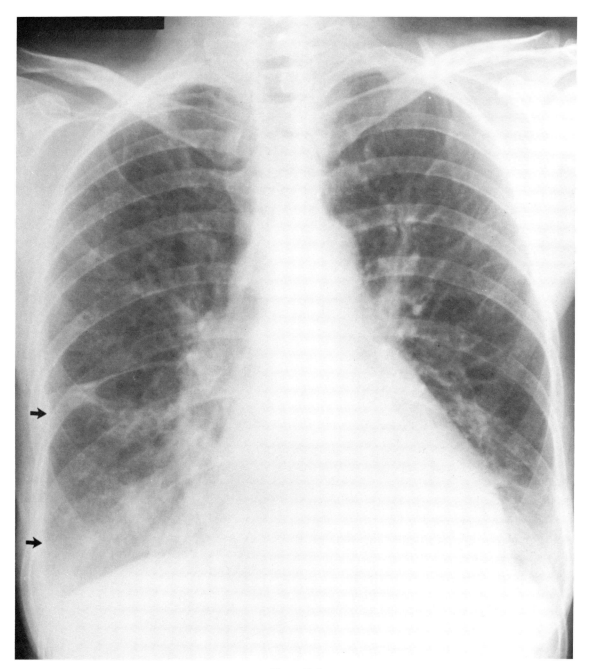

Figure C–3

Case C–3.   How does this patient differ from Case C–1?

DISCUSSION, CASE C–3

This patient was a 47 year old white female who presented with congestive heart failure. She had a chronic cardiac condition, in contrast to the
patient discussed in Case C–1. The radiograph shows edematous interstitial
septa (Kerley's B lines) and fluid collected inside the visceral pleura (in the
subpleural area) along the lateral chest wall (arrows). These two signs, which
are well-known and aid in the radiographic diagnosis of chronic congestive
heart failure, are important only if present. The absence of these signs does not
rule out congestive heart failure or pulmonary edema secondary to acute left
ventricular decompensation.

CASE C–4

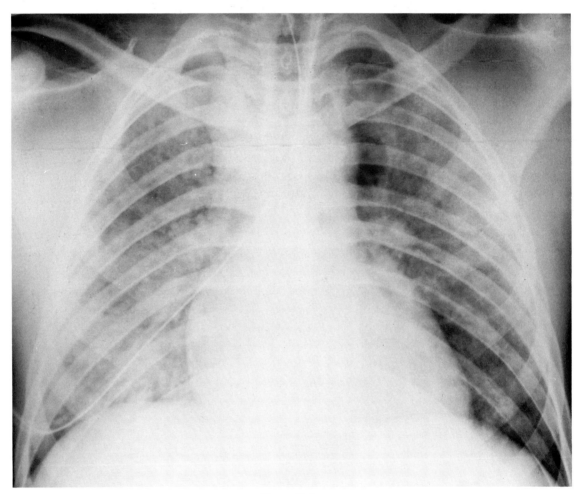

Figure C–4a

Case C–4a. This patient was a 27 year old white male who had been
stabbed in the right side of the neck. He had no other medical problems.
This radiograph (Fig. C–4a) was made immediately following surgical repair
of the neck laceration.

Figure C–4b

Case C –4b. Figure C–4b is a radiograph of the same patient in Figure
C–4a 6 days following surgery, at the time of discharge from the hospital.

DISCUSSION, CASE C–4

This patient clearly has pulmonary edema that is almost certainly caused by overhydration. Of course, one would have to know that the patient does not have a head injury or cardiac or renal failure and that there were no other surgical complications, before a definitive diagnosis of overhydration as the cause of the pulmonary edema could be made. An immediate conference with the patient's surgeons ascertained all the facts, and an adjustment of the patient's intravenous fluids led to complete elimination of his pulmonary edema within a few days.

CASE C–5

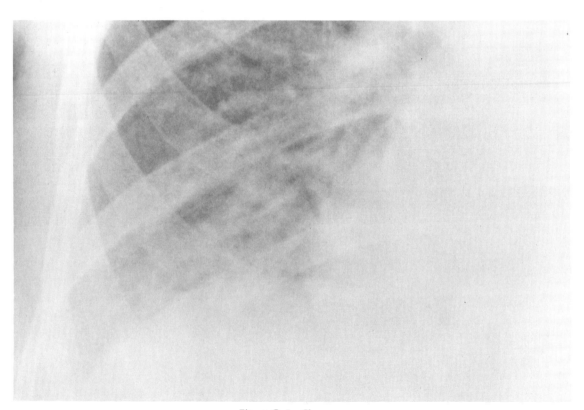

Figure C–5   Close-up

Figure C–5

Case C –5. This patient was a 45 year old white female who presented with increasing dyspnea and chest pain. She had a known chronic disease. What is your diagnostic evaluation of this patient's illness?

DISCUSSION, CASE C–5

The radiograph shows excess fluid in the lungs and in the pleural space. In addition, the patient has either cardiomegaly or a pericardial effusion. The radiographic findings are actually nonspecific, as they are compatible with congestive heart failure, uremic pneumonitis, and even lupus erythematosus. The known chronic disease, as I am sure you have guessed, is chronic renal failure. The radiograph demonstrates uremic pneumonitis, pericarditis with an effusion, and pleural effusion. One might legitimately ask whether the fluid in the lung represents hydrostatic edema or whether it is secondary to increased capillary permeability caused by the patient's known uremia. This question cannot be answered, and it is probable that both entities cause intraparenchymal fluid in patients with chronic renal failure, particularly in those who have cardiac manifestations of the disease.

CASE C–6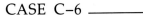

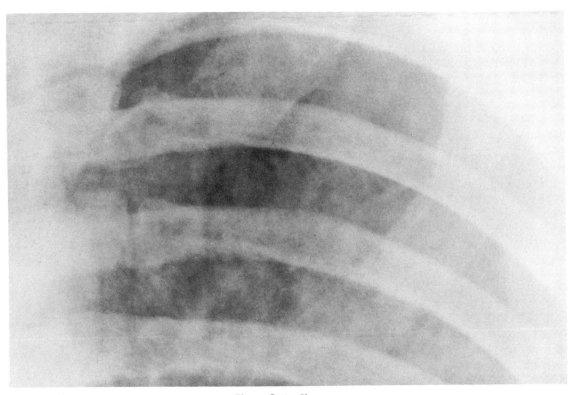

Figure C–6   Close-up

Figure C–6

Case C –6. This patient was a 25 year old white male who was brought to the emergency suite in an unconscious state. He had suffered no known trauma. This radiograph was made shortly after his arrival. What are the best possible diagnoses?

DISCUSSION, CASE C–6

Once again we have a radiographic picture of nonspecific pulmonary edema, and additional historical information is mandatory in order for us to arrive at a final conclusion. In cases such as this, physical examination almost always reveals evidence of chronic use of intravenous drugs, in this case, heroin.

CASE C–7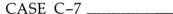

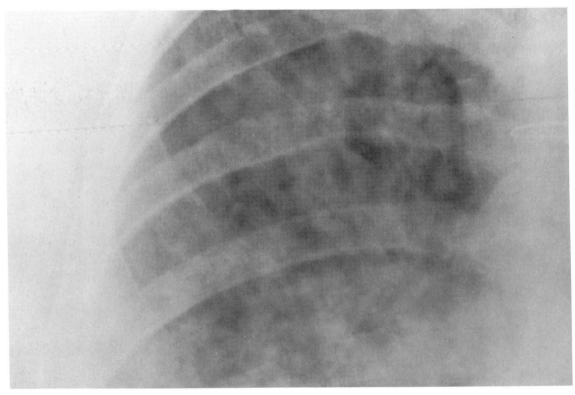

Figure C–7   Close-up

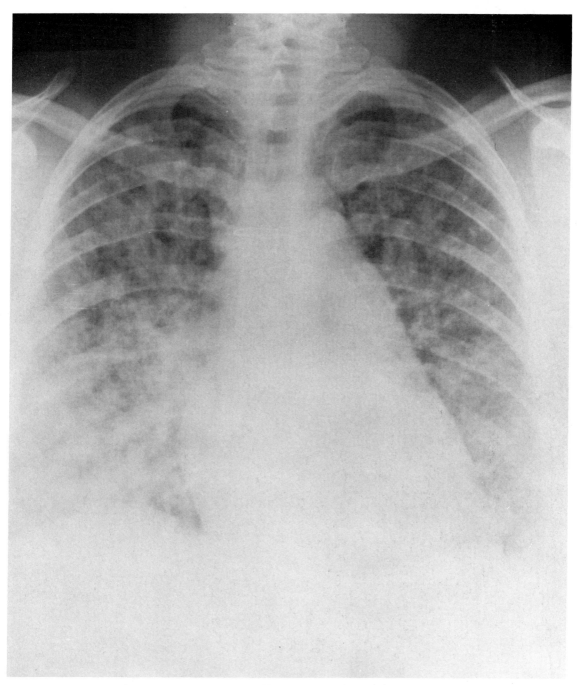

Figure C-7

Case C-7. This patient was a 45 year old white female who presented in the emergency suite with acute dyspnea. Approximately 2 hours before she presented, she had accidentally inhaled a considerable quantity of insecticide spray containing a hydrocarbon. Several years before, the patient had had replacement of a mitral valve, with an uneventful recovery and subsequent good health until this admission. What is your evaluation of this radiograph?

DISCUSSION, CASE C–7

The difference between this case of excess water in the lungs and the cases presented previously is immediately apparent. The distribution of the fluid is more peripheral than central and therefore represents a diffuse chemical pneumonitis. The mechanism, of course, is entirely different from that of hydrostatic pulmonary edema, and the distribution of the fluid is related to aspiration of the chemical to the periphery of the lungs. The patient's lungs were cleared of this pneumonitis within 48 hours, and she was discharged.

CASE C–8

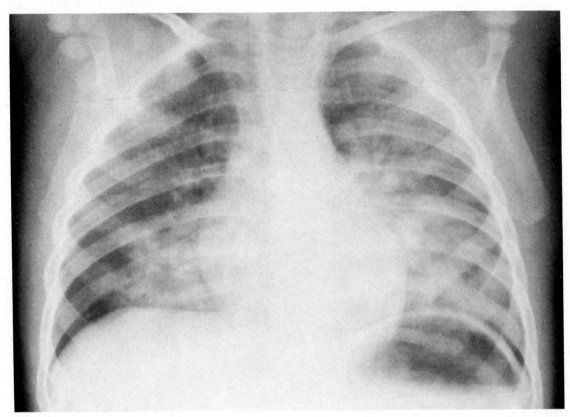

Figure C–8

Case C–8. This patient was a 14 month old white male who was brought to the emergency suite after having ingested and subsequently vomited a household cleaning agent containing a hydrocarbon. Compare this case with Case C–7. How do you think the cases are similar, and how do you think they differ?

DISCUSSION, CASE C–8

Note the difference between this chemical pneumonitis and that of the preceding case. This child aspirated the hydrocarbon and developed a bilateral aspiration chemical pneumonitis, in contrast to the preceding patient, who also inhaled a similar substance.

CASE C–9 _____

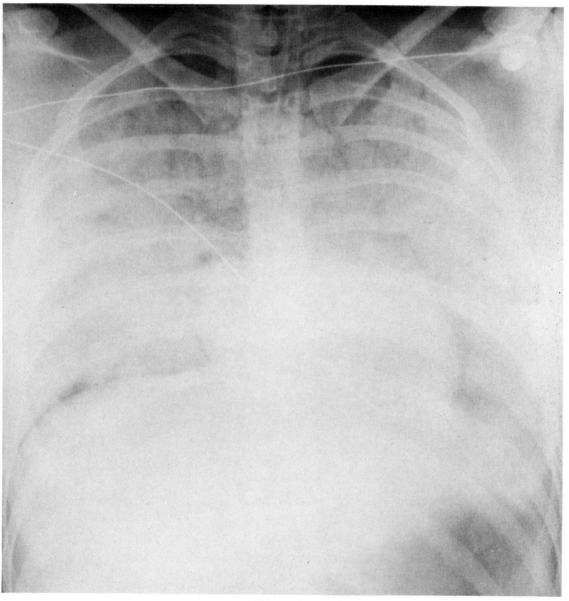

Figure C–9a

Case C –9a.   This patient was a 20 year old pregnant white female who presented with the onset of severe eclampsia. She was admitted in acute respiratory distress. A radiograph made several days later is seen on the next page.

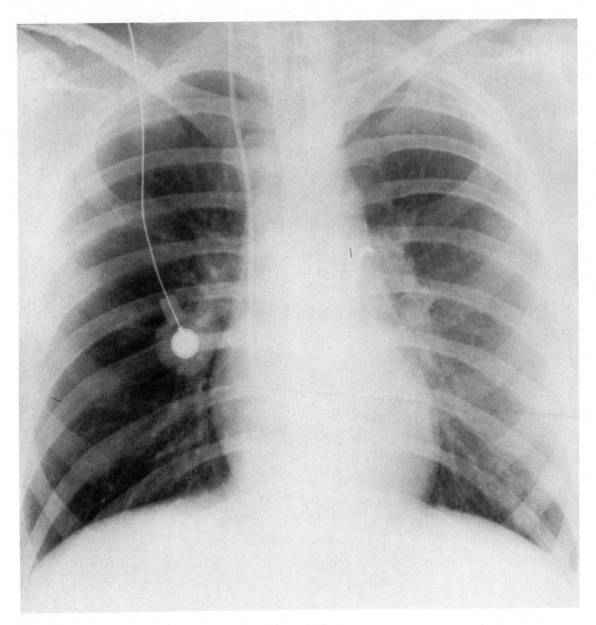

Figure C–9b

Case C–9b.   This radiograph of the same patient shown in Figure C–9a made 3 days after admission reveals complete clearance of the pulmonary edema. She had been placed on a respirator, but only moderate oxygen therapy was necessary.

This case and the three cases following it are in a certain sense related. All four will be discussed as a unit after Case C–12.

CASE C–10 _____

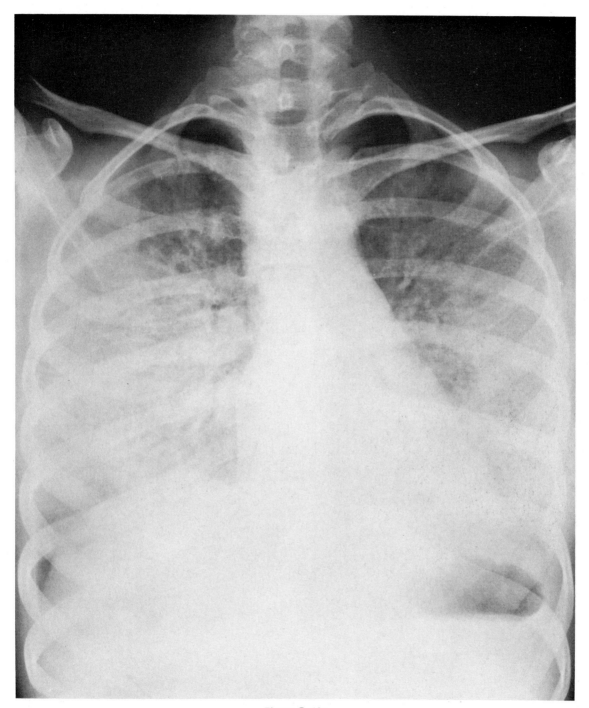

Figure C–10a

Case C –10a. This 17 year old white female was admitted to the hospital comatose and hypotensive after a drug overdose. She was placed on a respirator, and 100 per cent oxygen was necessary for approximately 14 hours.

A radiograph made several days later is seen on the next page.

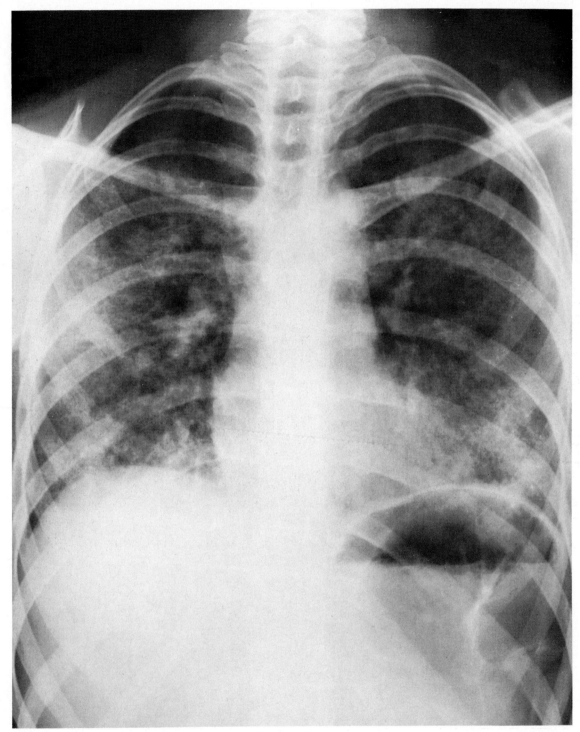

Figure C–10b

Case C –10b. This radiograph of the same patient shown in Figure C–10a was made 10 days after admission to the hospital. The patient's oxygen therapy was gradually decreased, but she was difficult to wean from the ventilator. She eventually recovered completely, however, and a chest radiograph made approximately 6 weeks after admission was clear.

CASE C–11 _____

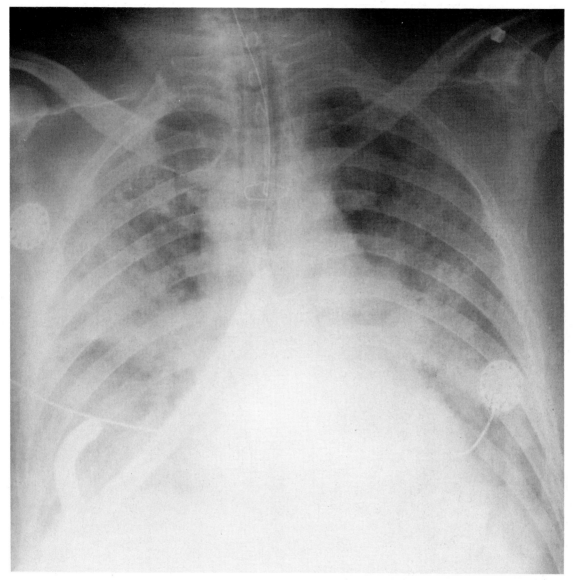

Figure C–11a

Case C–11a. This patient was a 52 year old white male who was well except for having coronary artery disease. This radiograph was made on the day following coronary bypass surgery, and it reveals postoperative pulmonary edema.

Two additional radiographs of this patient are on the next two pages.

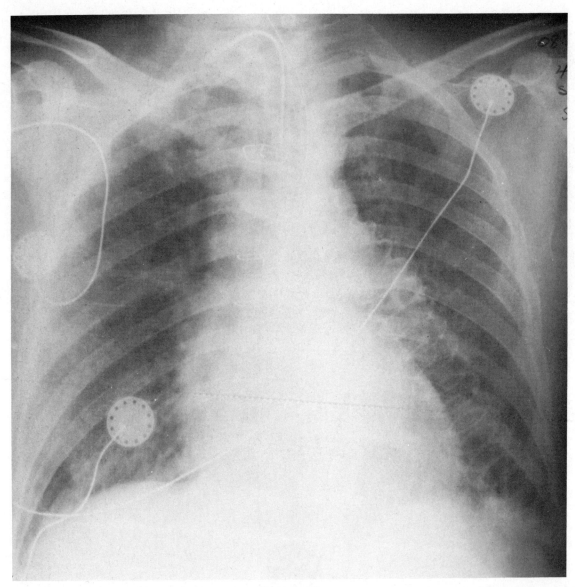

Figure C−11b

Case C−11b. This radiograph of the same patient shown in Figure C−11a was made 6 days later and reveals good clearance of the patient's pulmonary edema. A tracheostomy tube can be seen in place, and oxygen therapy was continued.

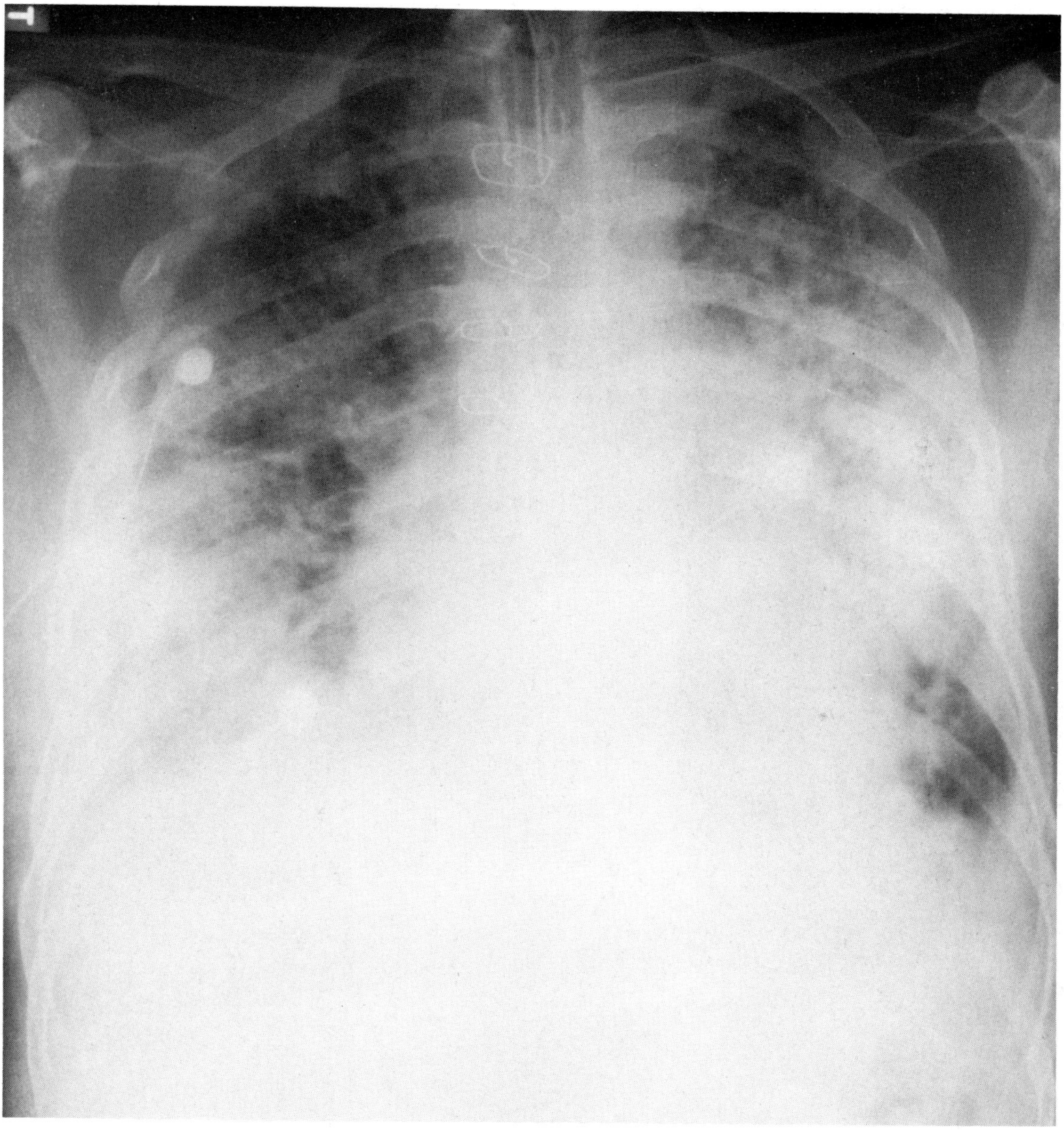

Figure C–11c

Case C–11c. This radiograph of the same patient shown in the last two figures was made 9 days after Figure C–11b and 16 days after surgery. Once again, there is diffuse pulmonary disease, but the character of these parenchymal changes is quite different from the character of the changes seen in Figure C–11a. After the patient was weaned from the respirator and oxygen therapy, he made a gradual recovery. At the time he was discharged from the hospital, however, residual pulmonary parenchymal changes were still present.

CASE C-12 _____

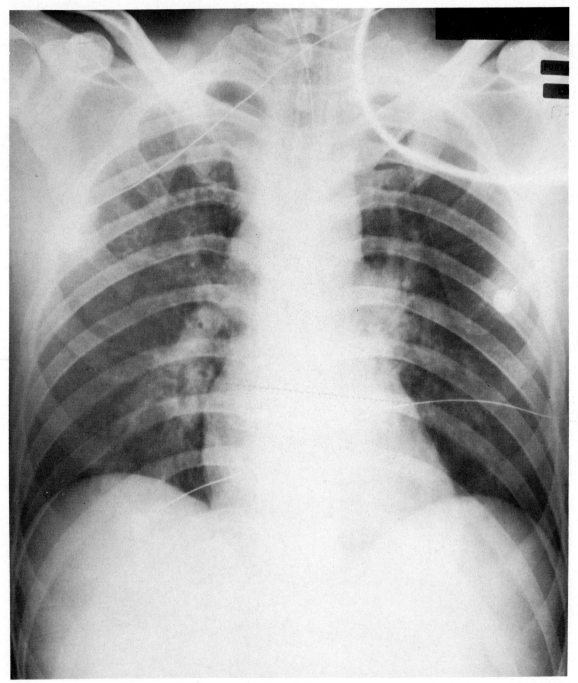

Figure C-12a

Case C-12a. This patient was a 44 year old white male who was admitted in a comatose condition secondary to a heat stroke. This radiograph was made on the day following admission.

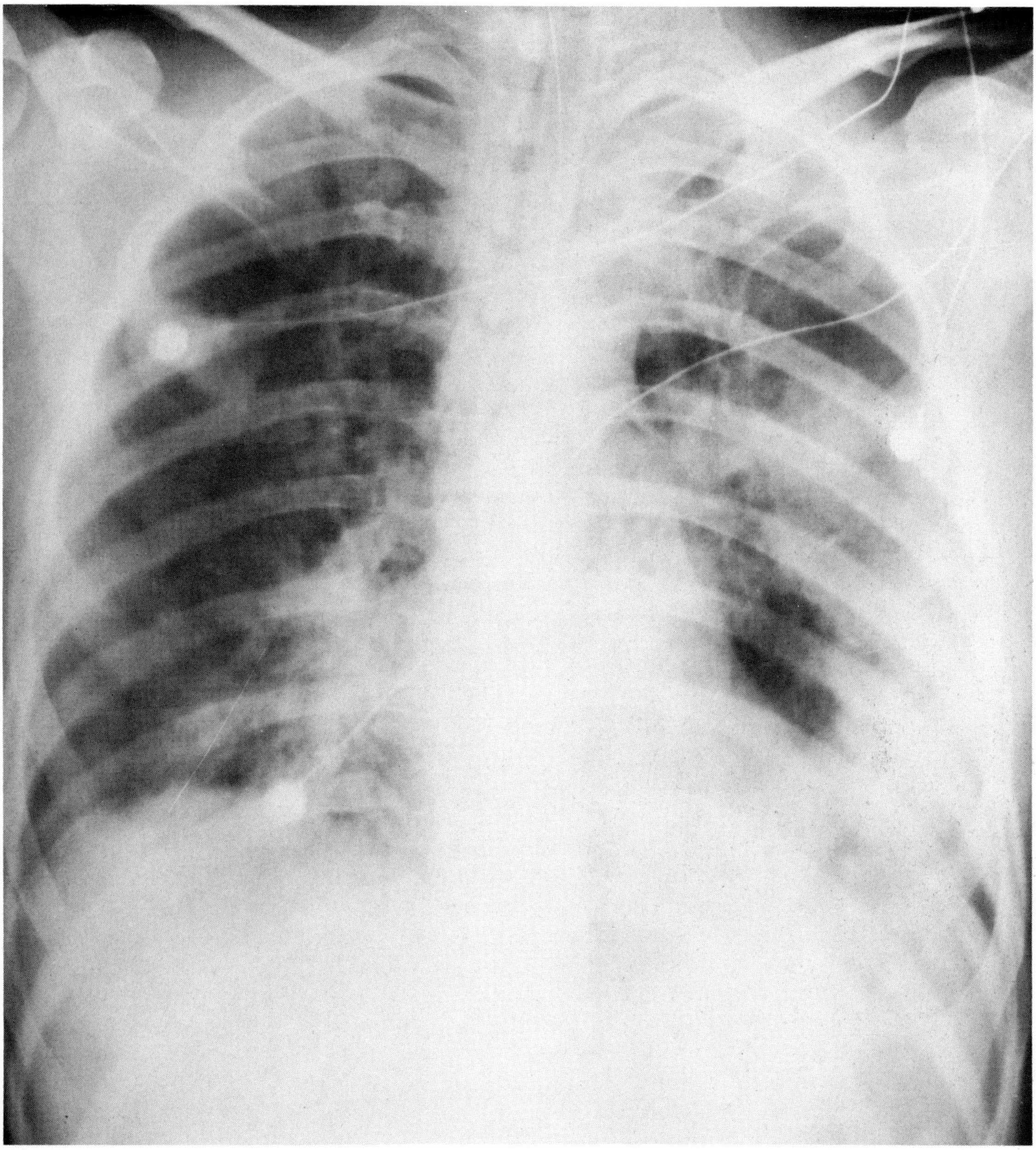

Figure C–12b

Case C –12b. This radiograph of the same patient shown in Figure C–12a was made on the third hospital day, and it demonstrates a bilateral airspace filling process. The patient died on the following day, and autopsy revealed massive pulmonary edema and hemorrhage. Disseminated intravascular coagulation (DIC) probably was present.

DISCUSSION, CASES C–9 through C–12

These four cases are related in that each patient had some degree of damage to the surfactant system and alteration of the permeability of the alveolocapillary membrane. However, the extent of the pathology varies from case to case. The first patient had pulmonary edema, evidently with minimal damage to the alveolocapillary membrane, and the water was cleared from her lungs in a very brief period of time. This is usually the case with hydrostatic pulmonary edema if the factors that were responsible for the initial development of the edema can be eliminated. However, the next three cases show varying degrees of damage to the alveolocapillary membrane and to the surfactant system. These patients have been grouped under the heading adult respiratory distress syndrome (ARDS). The pathological changes seen in the lungs at autopsy are related to the extent of damage to the alveolocapillary membrane and to the blood products that escape into the alveolar spaces. This damage leads to bronchopulmonary dysplasia and to the development of hyaline membranes — an oversimplified description of a complex process.

The list of causes of the adult respiratory distress syndrome is very long, and actually any disease process that can cause pulmonary edema can be placed on the list. Certainly any etiologic agent that can disrupt the surfactant system and increase alveolocapillary permeability must be on the list. Any patient who is admitted with nonhydrostatic pulmonary edema should be a suspect for the development of ARDS, particularly if oxygen therapy has been necessary. In the experience of this observer, oxygen therapy has been the most insidious and difficult to recognize cause of ARDS, and it has been quite difficult to determine the point at which the patient begins to develop ARDS. Oxygen therapy should be kept to a minimum, but high percentages of oxygen are often necessary to sustain the patient's life. The patient in Case C–11, however, is a case in point. All the pulmonary parenchymal changes after the first postoperative week were secondary to oxygen therapy and to the development of ARDS.

CASE C–13 _____

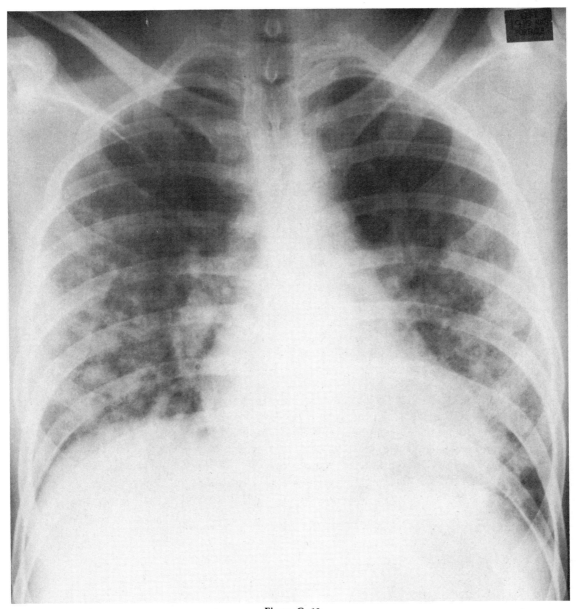

Figure C–13

Case C –13.   This patient was a 28 year old white male who was admitted to the hospital with multiple fractures following a motor vehicle accident. This radiograph was made approximately 36 hours following admission. Several possibilities should always be considered under the circumstances just described. What would you consider, and what is your best choice of diagnosis?

DISCUSSION, CASE C–13

Generally speaking, four possibilities must be considered with any patient who has suffered significant trauma. One of these is pulmonary edema secondary to a brain injury, another is aspiration pneumonitis, a third is pulmonary contusion or laceration, and a fourth is fat embolization. (Of course, only those traumatic events that might result in diffuse pulmonary disease are considered here. Disruption of the thoracic aorta, fracture of a bronchus, and other such entities are outside the scope of this text.) The four possibilities just noted can almost always be distinguished on the basis of the radiographic appearance and the clinical information. The patient shown in Figure C–13 fractured his femur and other bones and has multiple fat emboli. The changes in the patient's lung are actually secondary to chemical pneumonitis due to the breakdown of the fat into glycerol and fatty acids. The lungs of patients with this type of pneumonitis will generally clear spontaneously, but occasionally a moderate amount of supportive therapy is needed. Deaths caused by massive embolization have been reported.

CASE C–14 _____

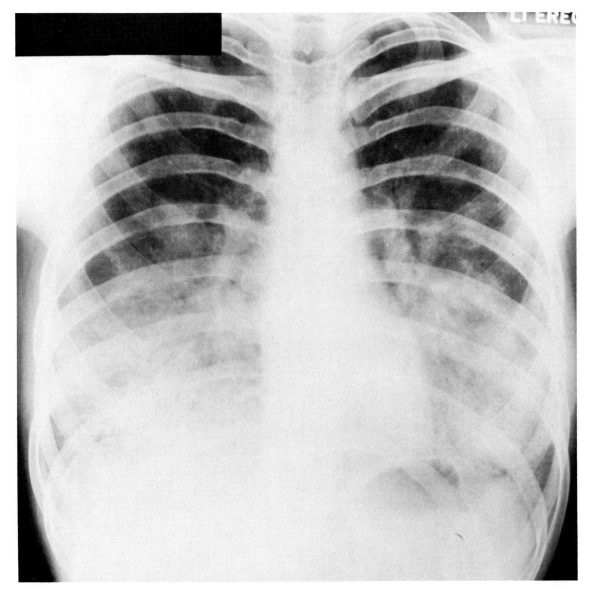

Figure C–14

Case C –14.   This patient was an 18 year old black female who presented with moderate dyspnea and a cough. What is your diagnosis?

DISCUSSION, CASE C–14

This radiograph shows considerable airspace filling, but the appearance of the radiograph does not correlate well with the clinical information. This single fact often leads to the correct diagnosis. Naturally, a careful history must be obtained to rule out inhalation of any toxic substance or a possible antigen-antibody reaction. However, those patients who have either of these problems are invariably more symptomatic. The virtual absence of symptomatology relative to the pronounced airspace filling seen in the radiograph allows us in this case to diagnose alveolar proteinosis. This is an unusual and interesting entity. The cause of the deposition of the lipoproteinaceous material in the airspaces is in some way related to excess surfactant, but the etiology of the disease certainly has not been clarified. The majority of patients who develop alveolar proteinosis recover spontaneously, although the condition can recur. Some patients, however, develop a superimposed infection, and one of the most common organisms to occur in these patients is *Nocardia*. Recent work has shown a relationship between alveolar proteinosis, the hematologic malignancies, and lymphoma.

CASE C-15 _____

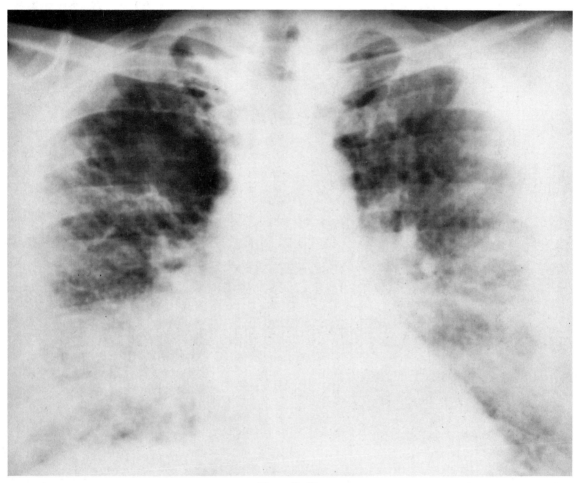

Figure C-15a

Case C-15a. This patient was a 50 year old male who presented as an emergency case with acute dyspnea. He had been well except for a moderate chronic cough and occasional dyspnea on exertion What kind of alveolar filling process do you think this patient has? Why is it asymmetric?

Try to make the diagnosis before looking on the next page at a radiograph of the same patient made 1 week later.

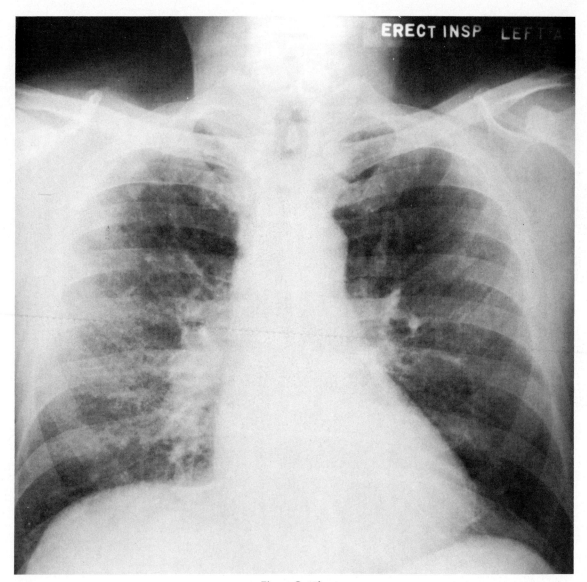

Figure C–15b

Case C –15b   This radiograph was made of the same patient shown in Figure C–15a 1 week following admission after appropriate therapy.

DISCUSSION, CASE C–15

If you made the diagnosis of acute pulmonary edema you are correct, but how can we account for the pronounced asymmetry? The patient had long-standing obstructive airways disease, but it is much more marked in some areas than in others. We can tell by the distribution of pulmonary edema that the patient's best remaining vascular bed is in his right lower lobe. The right upper lobe, on the other hand, is most affected by the patient's obliterative pulmonary vascular changes. Naturally, gravity may account for some of the distribution of the pulmonary edema. However, if we observe the radiograph made 1 week after appropriate therapy, we see that the vasculature in the right lower lobe is considerably more abundant than that in the right upper lobe and that that in the left lung is of intermediate abundance. This asymmetric or regional distribution of pulmonary edema is not uncommon and must be expected in patients with obstructive airways disease. Of the four patterns of edema described by Hublitz and Shapiro,[6] this observer has found the regional pattern to be by far the most common.

REFERENCES

1. Carnovale, R., Zornoza, J., Goldman, A. M., et al.: Pulmonary alveolar proteinosis: its association with hematologic malignancy and lymphoma. Radiology, 122:303–306, 1977.
2. Don, C., and Johnson, R.: The nature and significance of peribronchial cuffing in pulmonary edema. Radiology, 125:577–582, 1977.
3. Dyck, D. R., and Zylak, C. J.: Acute respiratory distress in adults. Radiology, 106:497–501, 1973.
4. Fraser, R. G., and Paré, J. A. P.: Diagnosis of Diseases of the Chest, 2nd ed. Philadelphia, W. B. Saunders Co., 1977.
5. Heitzman, E. R.: The Lung: Radiologic and Pathologic Correlations. St. Louis, C. V. Mosby Co., 1973.
6. Hublitz, U. F., and Shapiro, J. H.: Atypical pulmonary patterns of congestive failure in chronic lung disease. Radiology, 93:995–1006, 1969.
7. Joffe, N.: The adult respiratory distress syndrome. Am. J. Roentgenol., 122:719–732, 1974.
8. Milne, E. N. C.: Correlation of physiologic findings with chest roentgenology. Radiol. Clin. North Am., 12(1):17–47, 1973.
9. Pitt, M. J., and Freundlich, I. M.: Shifting pulmonary edema. Unpublished data.
10. Robin, E. D., Cross, C. E., and Zelis, R.: Pulmonary edema. N. Engl. J. Med., 288(5):239–246, 1973.
11. Robin, E. D., Cross, C. E., and Zelis, R.: Pulmonary edema. N. Engl. J. Med., 288(6):292–304, 1973.

Is pulmonary hyperaeration and/or
pulmonary arterial hypertension the
dominant feature?

Section D

If the answers to the first three diagnostic questions of Sections A, B, and C are no, then one should consider whether pulmonary hyperaeration and/or pulmonary arterial hypertension is the dominant feature. It is usually not difficult to determine that a patient has primary airways obstructive disease, rather than compensatory, secondary hyperaeration. Although many end-stage pulmonary diseases exhibit bronchiectasis, cystic bronchiolectasis (honeycombing), and compensatory hyperaeration, the secondary nature of these obstructive changes is usually easily established.

The problem in this section will be to attempt to decide which of the airways obstructive diseases or combinations thereof is the most likely diagnosis. The following are the various types of airways obstructive diseases:

1. Emphysema
   a. Panacinar emphysema (type A)
   b. Centrilobular emphysema (type B)
   c. Alpha-1 antitrypsin deficiency
   d. Bullous emphysema
2. Asthma
3. Chronic infection of airways
   a. Chronic bronchitis
   b. Bronchiectasis
   c. Cystic fibrosis

Decision 1. Does the patient have emphysema?

PANACINAR EMPHYSEMA (TYPE A), CENTRILOBULAR EMPHYSEMA (TYPE B). Generalized emphysema can be divided into the preceding two types, although this division is undoubtedly an oversimplification. The patient with panacinar emphysema is the typical "pink puffer," who in the later stages of his illness is barrel-chested, wasted, and markedly dyspneic. Pulmonary arterial hypertension and cor pulmonale are relatively late manifestations. The patient with centrilobular emphysema, which is frequently associated with chronic bronchitis, is most often the edematous "blue-bloater," who has a chronic productive cough as well as considerable shortness of breath. From the radiographic standpoint the latter type of emphysematous patient appears to be more normal but is actually just as ill clinically. The development of pulmonary arterial hypertension is apparently more rapid in centrilobular emphysema, and may indeed be the earliest definitive radiographic manifestation of the patient's illness. (*Note:* Pulmonary arterial hypertension may occur secondary to a number of disease entities, which fit into the following three general categories:

1. obstruction within the left side of the heart, usually caused by mitral stenosis, rarely by a myxoma;
2. left to right intracardiac or extracardiac shunts; and
3. primary-pulmonary disease, which includes
   a. obliterative pulmonary vascular disease,
   b. multiple pulmonary emboli or schistosomiasis, and
   c. idiopathic pulmonary hypertension.)

The term chronic obstructive pulmonary (lung) disease (COPD or COLD) includes patients with types A and B emphysema (panacinar and centrilobular). A third group, however, whose obstructive airways disease and chronic bronchitis involve the smallest bronchi rather than the major ones is also included. The patients of this group may actually merit a separate classification, as they do not fit well into COPD type A or type B. They are different in that their airways obstructive disease, involving the smallest bronchi, is exceedingly difficult to measure by the routine pulmonary function tests. The radiographs are always virtually normal until the later stages, and these patients represent a difficult group to manage. The term COPD, however, has been broadened to include all types of airways obstructive disease, with or without chronic infection.

It must be kept in mind that if patients with chronic obstructive lung disease suffer left ventricular failure, the appearance of the interstitial and even the alveolar edema will be atypical, as we saw in the previous section. In a patient with known *obstructive disease and acute dyspnea* the possibility of *left ventricular heart failure* should always be given *primary consideration.*

The following are the two remaining types of emphysema.

    c. Alpha-1 antitrypsin deficiency— The individual carrying the homozygous form of this inborn enzyme deficiency usually presents with lower lobe hyperaeration as the first sign of a significant emphysematous process.
    d. Bullous emphysema

Decision 2. Does the patient have asthma? Asthmatic patients have airways obstruction but are not usually included in the differential diagnosis of diffuse pulmonary disease. However, one condition, allergic aspergillosis, which is almost always found in asthmatic patients or in those with cystic fibrosis, must be kept in mind. In this entity, mucus plugs that contain the mycelia of *Aspergillus* are found in dilated middle order bronchi. There may be distal pneumonitis or atelectasis, or both, associated with the plugging of these bronchi. (Asthma will also be considered with the hypersensitivity reactions in Section E.)

Decision 3. Does the patient have a chronic airways infection?

CHRONIC BRONCHITIS — A CHRONIC PRODUCTIVE COUGH

BRONCHIECTASIS. This entity, which consists of fusiform, cylindrical, or sacular dilatation of airways, is due to chronic infection in the walls of the bronchi. It is at times a local disease, but it may also be a generalized process that is part of an overall airways obstructive picture. The bronchiectatic cysts may be seen on plain radiographs only if the cysts are large enough or if the walls are considerably thickened. Bronchiectatic cysts often become obvious when there is surrounding superimposed pneumonitis. However, this entity must be differentiated from necrotizing pneumonia with early cavitation.

CYSTIC FIBROSIS. This congenital enzymatic abnormality is usually discovered in infancy or early childhood, but occasionally cases do not come to light until adolescence or even early adult life. The radiologic picture is usually typical and consists of

    a. hyperaeration
    b. thickened peribronchial soft tissues or bronchial walls
    c. distal areas of chronic infection or atelectasis, or both

(*Note:* Thickened peribronchial soft tissues have been described in multiple entities. Any local inflammatory condition may cause edematous thickened peribronchial soft tissues in the affected portion of lung, but in the case of generalized pulmonary disease, this particular finding can be divided into acute and chronic conditions. The acute conditions with thickened peribronchial soft tissues or bronchial walls are asthma and interstitial pulmonary edema; the chronic, cystic fibrosis and chronic bronchitis.)

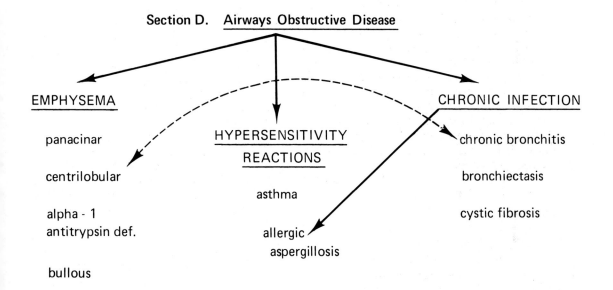

Section D. Airways Obstructive Disease

EMPHYSEMA

panacinar

centrilobular

alpha - 1
antitrypsin def.

bullous

HYPERSENSITIVITY
REACTIONS

asthma

allergic
aspergillosis

CHRONIC INFECTION

chronic bronchitis

bronchiectasis

cystic fibrosis

(pulmonary edema may be superimposed)

Figure D

CASE D–1 _____

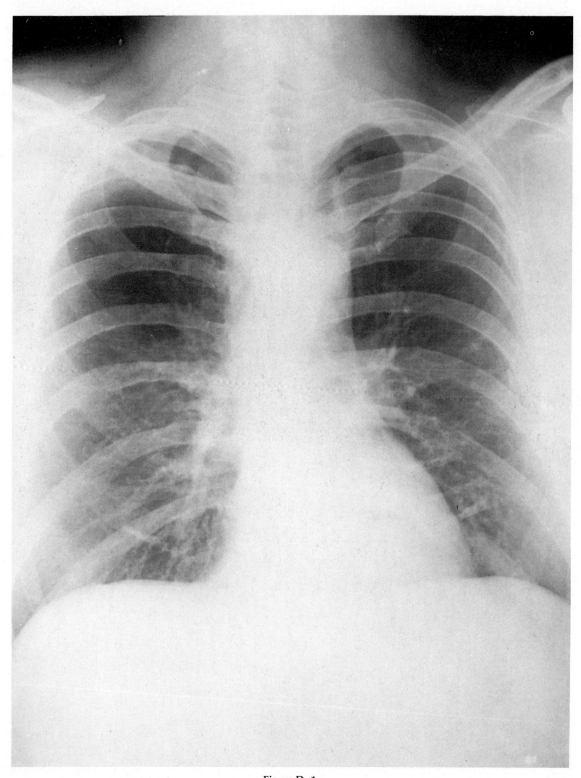

Figure D–1a

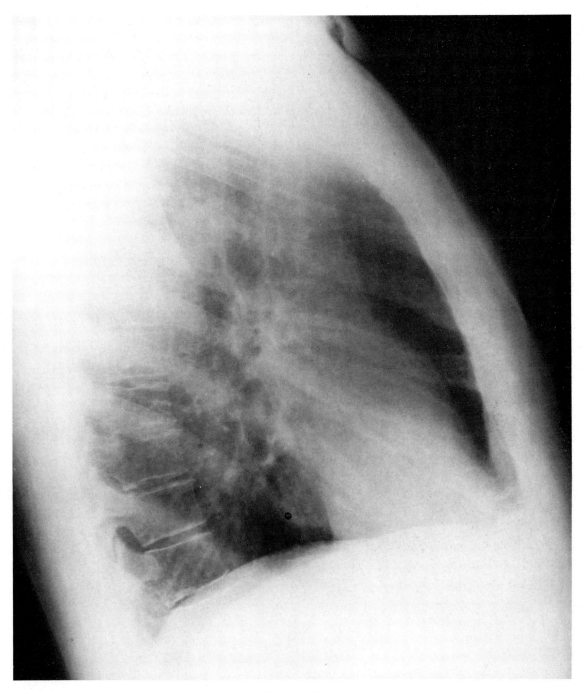

Figure D–1b

Case D–1a and D–1b. This patient was a 37 year old white male who complained only of minimal dyspnea on exertion. Would you call this chest (Figs. D–1a and D–1b) normal or abnormal? Additional radiographs of this patient will be found on the next two pages. Discussion of Case D–1 will be found on page 146.

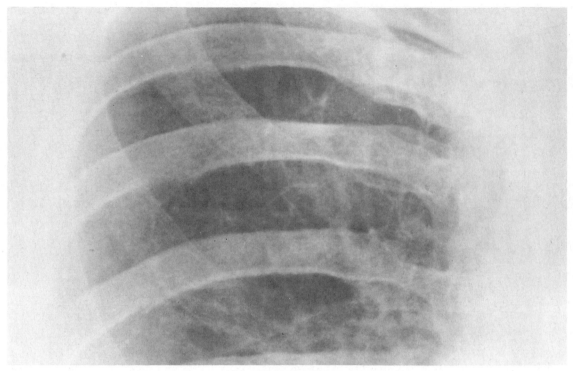

Figure D–1c

Case D–1c and D–1d.   Figure D–1c above is a close-up of the patient's right upper lobe. Compare it with Figure D–1d below, which is a close-up of the right upper lobe of an entirely normal patient.

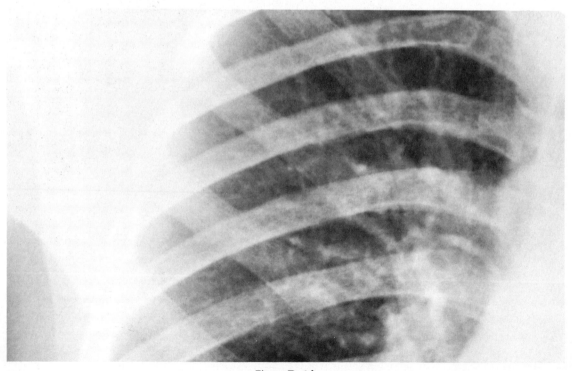

Figure D–1d

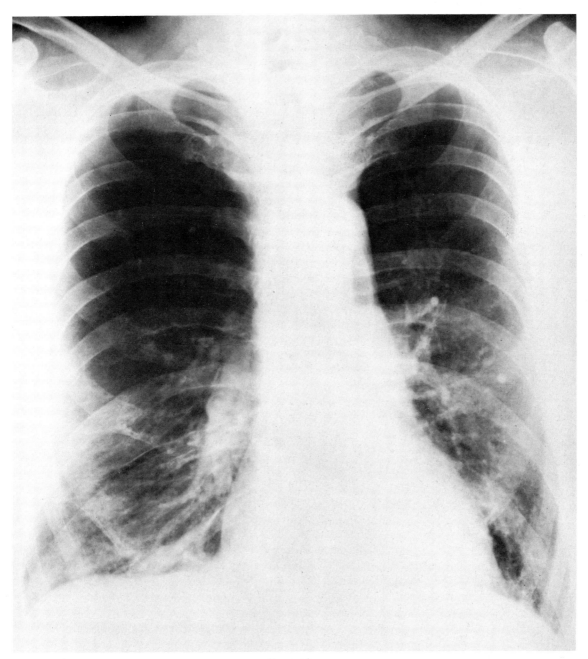

Figure D–1e

Case D–1e. Figure D–1e is a radiograph of the same patient shown in Figures D–1a, b, and c 15 years later.

DISCUSSION, CASE D-1

There are probably some radiologists who would call the radiographs of Figures D-1a and D-1b within normal limits. Actually, the patient had moderately advanced upper lobe emphysema. Unfortunately, a chest radiograph can detect emphysematous changes only if they are moderately advanced. Thus far, early emphysema cannot be detected by routine chest radiography. However, diagnosis of emphysema at its earliest stage is of considerable importance to many patients, for if they can be induced to stop smoking, their lives can be significantly prolonged. Therefore, it is incorrect to call the radiographs of Figures D-1a and D-1b within normal limits, even if a comment about the upper lobe hyperaeration is included. In my opinion, the radiologic diagnosis should indicate that there are moderately advanced upper lobe changes compatible with a diagnosis of emphysema. (There are those clinicians who claim that radiologists should not diagnose emphysema, as not all hyperaeration is due to emphysema. A radiologist should give his opinion of which disease best fits the radiologic findings; this is just as true for emphysema as it would be for an ulcerating gastric lesion or a renal mass. Obviously, emphysema is not the only cause of hyperaeration, but it is of overriding importance to alert the clinician to the possibility of emphysema, even though the hyperaeration in some cases may be caused by something else.)

The recognition of a hyperaerated emphysematous chest should not depend upon the radiographic density of the lungs, as it is clear that this can be altered by changing technique. The best sign of emphysema within a single lobe or within multiple lobes is the altered appearance of the pulmonary vasculature. A comparison of Figures D-1c and D-1d will demonstrate this change very clearly. Note also the depression of the hilar arteries in Figure D-1a. To these findings can be added the moderately increased anterior airspace on the lateral view and the moderate flattening of the diaphragm. It should also be borne in mind that generalized pulmonary hyperaeration can often be observed in all three dimensions, cranio-caudad, anterior-posterior, and medial-lateral. The medial-lateral overexpansion causes the hilar arteries to be prominent in any hyperaerated chest. However, as the airways obstructive disease progresses there is obliteration of the peripheral pulmonary vascular bed, and the hilar arteries and the main pulmonary artery may demonstrate pulmonary hypertension.

In Figure D-1e the heart is considerably larger than expected in this emphysematous patient, indicating cardiac decompensation.

CASE D-2 _____

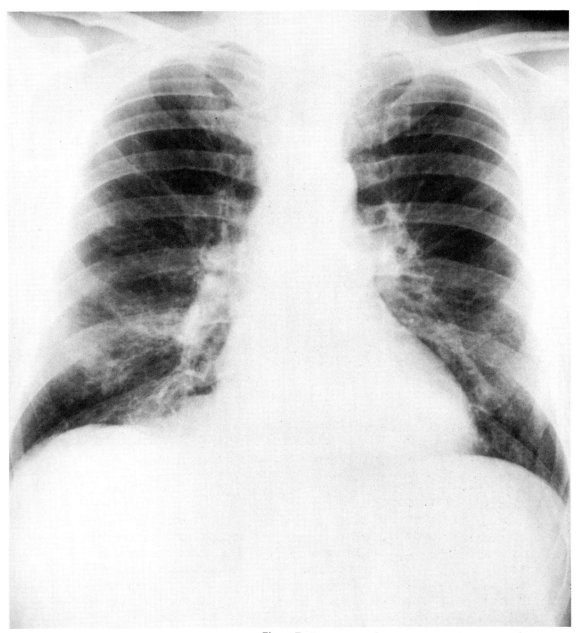

Figure D-2a

Case D-2a. This patient was a 53 year old white male who presented with a chronic productive cough and moderate shortness of breath. Would you call this chest normal or abnormal? A later radiograph of the same patient will be found on the next two pages.

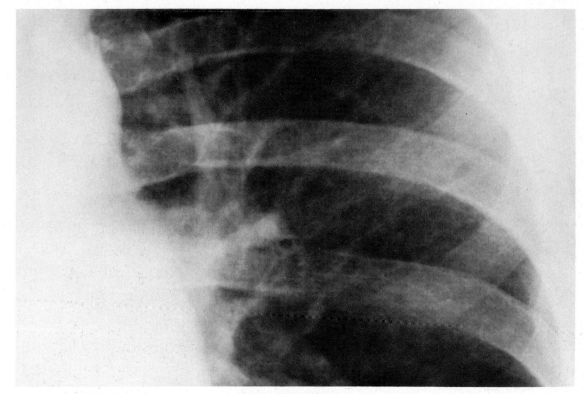

Figure D–2b   Close-up

DISCUSSION, CASE D–2

Although the patient seen in Figure D–2a already had significant pulmonary emphysema, it is even harder to recognize than the emphysema noted in Figure D–1a. A moderate attenuation of the vessels in the left upper lobe can be noted, and perhaps the main pulmonary artery and hilar arteries are somewhat larger than they should be, but otherwise the chest is relatively normal in appearance for a 53 year old male. However, it is clear in retrospect that he had emphysema, clinical chronic bronchitis, and pulmonary arterial hypertension at the time that the initial radiograph was made. The changes are much more severe 4 years later; the patient has marked pulmonary arterial hypertension and is a respiratory cripple.

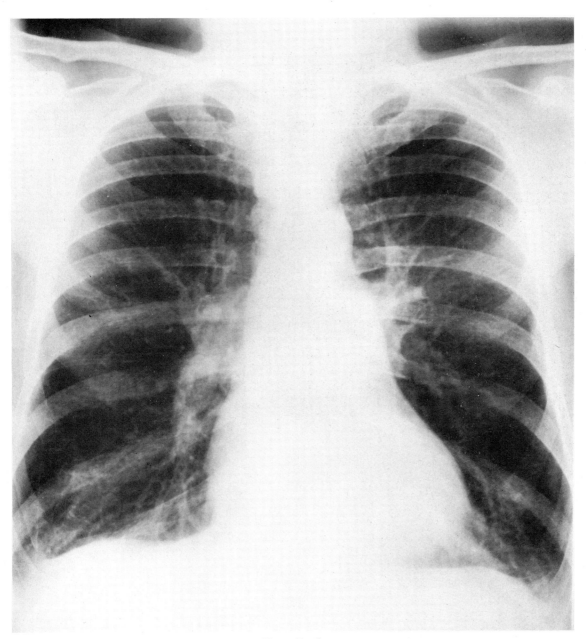

Figure D–2b

Case D–2b.   This is a radiograph of the same patient 4 years later. Note the marked changes that occurred in a relatively short period of time.

CASE D–3

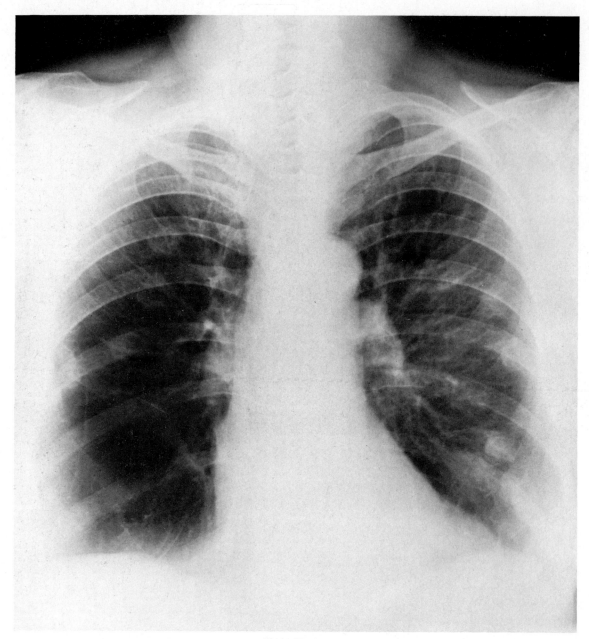

Figure D–3a

Case D–3a and D–3b. This patient was a 47 year old white female who presented with moderately increasing dyspnea. The patient had multiple healed rib fractures and a partially collapsed thoracic vertebra secondary to an old injury. What is your opinion of this patient's chest?

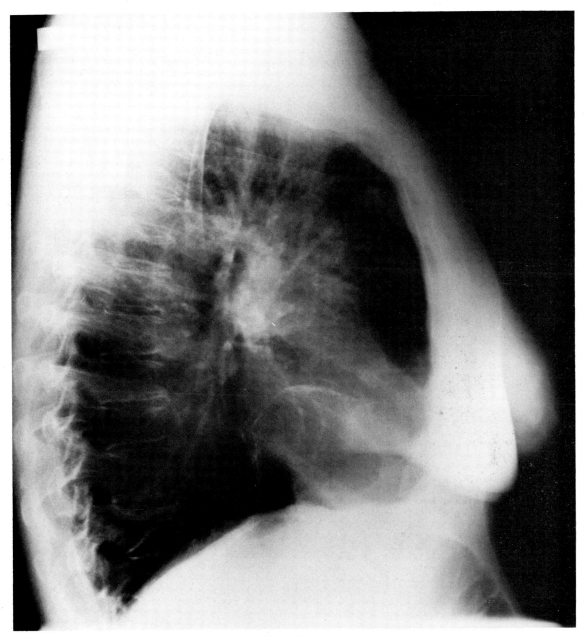

Figure D–3b

DISCUSSION, CASE D–3

This patient's emphysema is secondary to an alpha-1 antitrypsin deficiency. The typical radiologic change in this type of emphysema is a bilateral
lower lobe hyperaeration generally found in relatively young male patients.
However, recently, homozygous alpha-1 antitrypsin deficiency has been described in patients with various kinds of emphysema and has also been
found in children with chronic obstructive airways disease.

This particular patient probably had had emphysema for a number of
years and is somewhat atypical in that the changes in the right lower lobe
are more bullous than generalized.

CASE D–4 _____

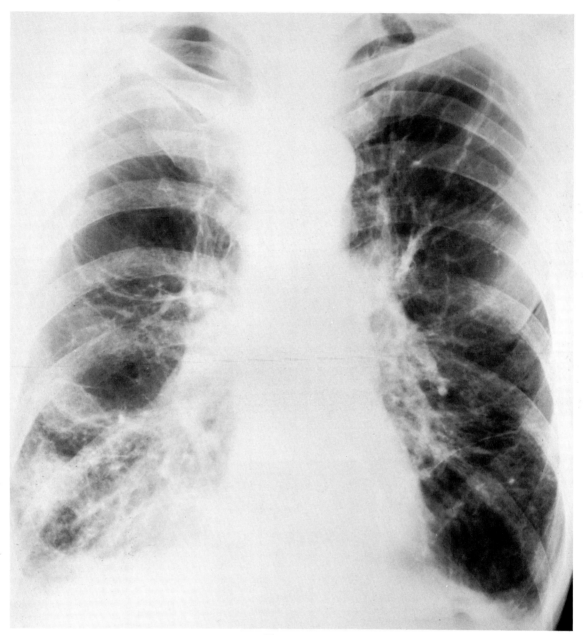

Figure D–4a

Case D–4a. This patient was a 68 year old white male with known chronic lung disease who presented with fever, a productive cough, and an increase in his dyspnea. An earlier radiograph of this patient is shown on the next page.

Figure D–4b

Case D–4b. This is a radiograph of the same patient shown in Figure D–4a 3 weeks earlier. Cases D–4 and D–5 are similar and will be discussed as a unit on page 156.

CASE D–5 _____

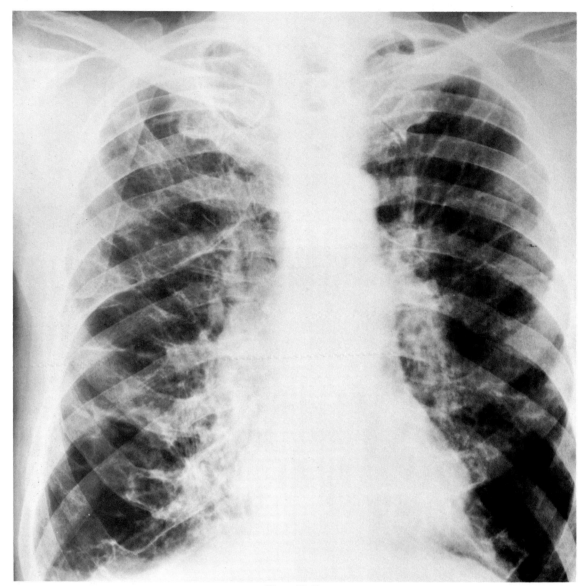

Figure D–5a

Case D–5a.   This was a 75 year old white male with known chronic lung disease who presented with fever, a productive cough, and an increase in his dyspnea. A radiograph made 2 days later is shown on the next page.

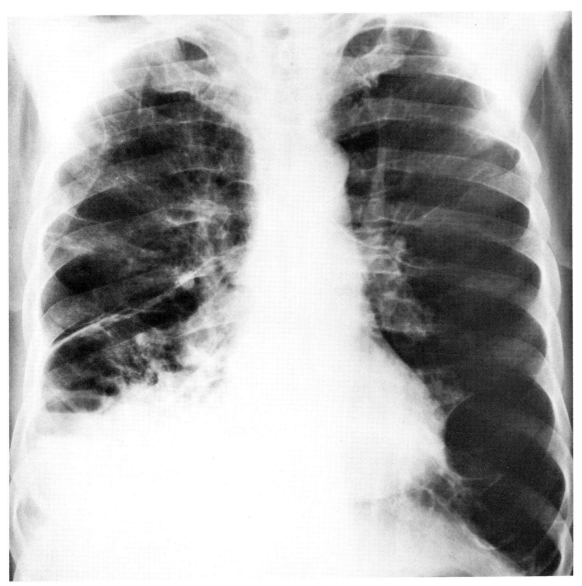

Figure D–5b

Case D–5b. This is a radiograph of the same patient shown in Figure D–5a 2 days later.

DISCUSSION, CASES D–4 and D–5

The patients shown in Figures D–4 and D–5 have many manifestations of chronic obstructive airways disease and chronic pulmonary infection. Both have bullous emphysema as well. The bullae in Figure D–4a are clearly obvious, and the patient has developed pneumonitis in his relatively normal right lower lobe. Having the old radiograph to compare to Figure D–4a makes the diagnosis obvious, with only the alternate possibility of superimposed pulmonary edema to be considered. Without the previous radiograph, however, it certainly would have been difficult to ascertain whether the disease in the right lower lobe was old or new.

The patient shown in Figure D–5 clearly has marked airways obstructive disease, but the bullae are not as easily seen as those in Figure D–4. However, 2 days following his admission to the hospital multiple bullae in the right lower lobe are obvious because of the air-fluid levels. As far as differential diagnosis is concerned, one must consider the possibility of empyema and a bronchopleural fistula. Patients with bullous emphysema or other chronic obstructive airways diseases always have a high risk of superimposed infection. Bullae will demonstrate air-fluid levels if they participate in the infection.

The heart is typically narrow and elongated in emphysematous patients (Fig. D–4a), and a heart that does not have this appearance in spite of significant emphysema should make one suspicious of cardiac decompensation.

CASE D–6

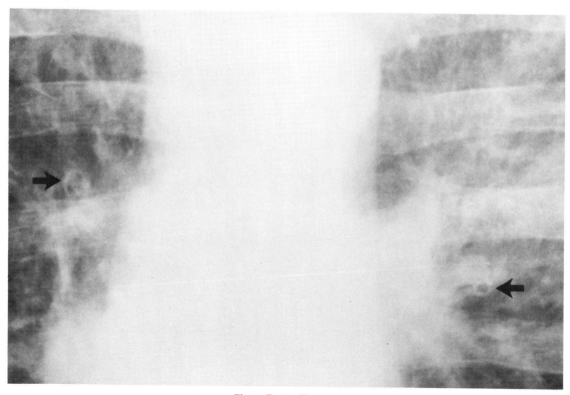

Figure D–6 Close-up

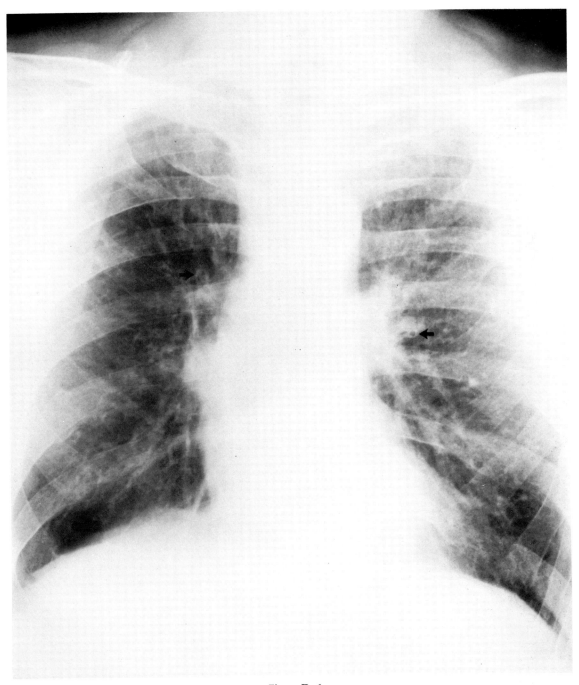

Figure D–6

Case D–6. This patient was a 64 year old white male who presented with a chronic productive cough and moderate dyspnea on exertion. What should the radiologist report in this type of case?

DISCUSSION, CASE D-6

This patient has chronic bronchitis and emphysema. Significant chronic bronchitis may not be appreciated radiographically at all, although in some patients thickened and irregular bronchial walls (arrows) may help confirm the diagnosis. To make such a diagnosis, the radiologist would have to know that the patient is not acutely dyspneic, as similar changes can be seen in early interstitial pulmonary edema. The difference in density between the two lungs is secondary to marked attenuation of the pulmonary blood flow through the right lung, in contrast to the more normal left side.

CASE D-7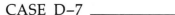

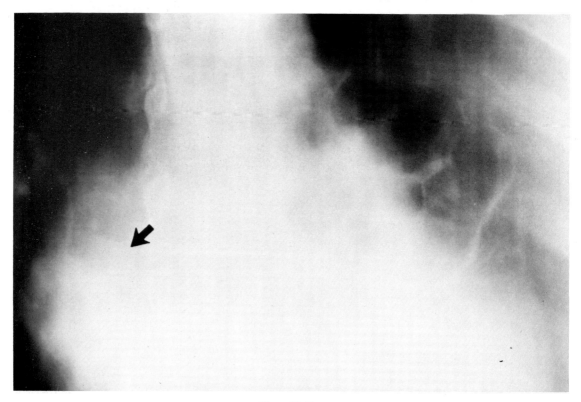

Figure D-7a

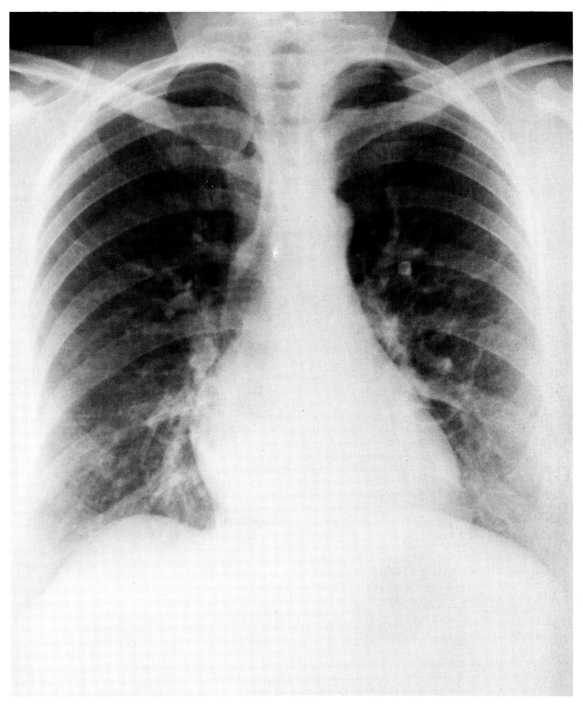

Figure D-7b

Case D-7a and D-7b. This patient was a 40 year old white female who presented with hemoptysis. Her past history is of interest in that she had had three previous episodes of pneumonia that cleared when she received antibiotic therapy, and previously she had had hemoptysis with pregnancies. The close-up (Fig. D-7a) is a tomogram made 3 days after the admission chest radiograph (Fig. D-7b). What kind of disease do you think this patient had, and what do you think the mass-like density in the right lung represents (arrowhead)? A bronchogram of the same patient is shown on the next two pages.

CASE D–7 *CONTINUED*

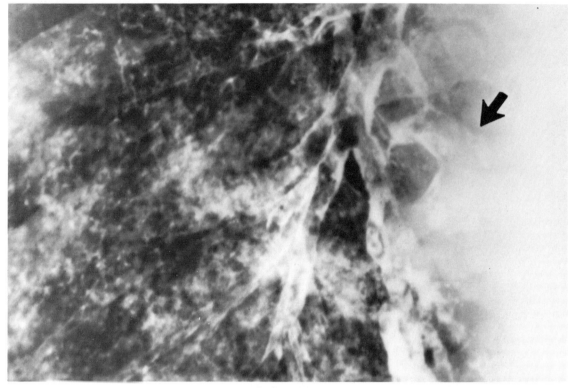

Figure D–7c

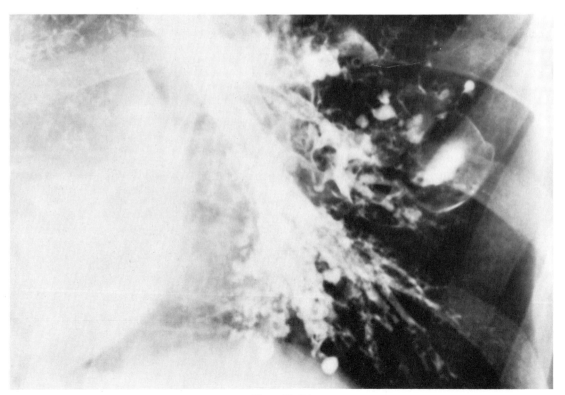

Figure D–7d

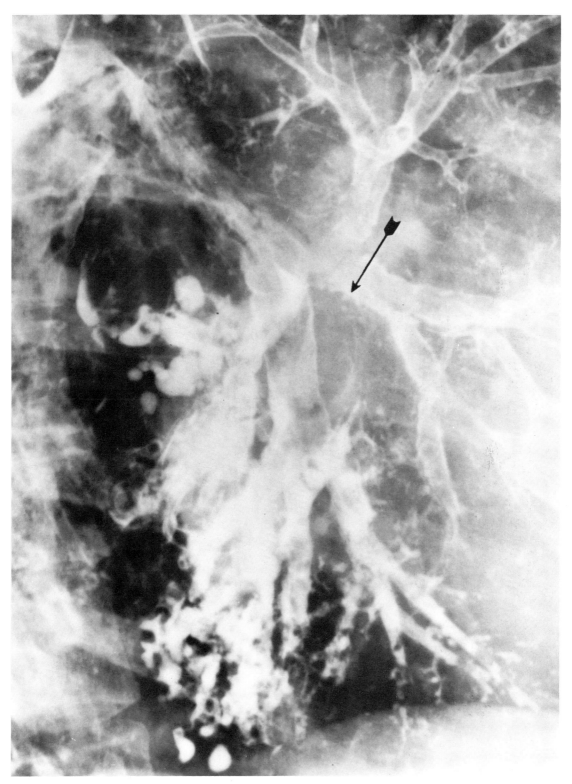

Figure D–7e

Case D–7c, d, and e.   Figures D–7c, d, and e are from a bronchogram made 5 days after admission. Figure D–7c shows the right lower chest, and Figures D–7d and e show the left lung. Incidentally, this bronchogram was made without any sort of intubation or instrumentation.[7]

DISCUSSION, CASE D-7

This patient had bronchiectasis, and the recognition of this disease on the basis of plain radiographs depends entirely upon the degree of bronchial dilatation. Minimal fusiform bronchiectasis generally will not be visible on plain radiographs of the chest, but as the dilated bronchi become larger and cylindrical or saccular, as in this case, the diagnosis is easily recognized. The impaction of one or more of the bronchiectatic sacs (arrowhead, Fig. D-7a), however, may suggest the erroneous diagnosis of a mass lesion, unless other similar but air-filled sacs can be seen. The arrowhead on Figure D-7c shows a dilated bronchus coated with contrast material, but very minimal contrast appears in the large sac in the right lower lobe because of the inspissated material already present within it. The tailed arrow on Figure D-7e demonstrates one of many distended mucus glands that are secondary to chronic bronchitis and are now filled with contrast material.

It is important for the radiologist to recognize that the patient has moderate but very extensive bronchiectasis throughout both lower lobes. None of the lower lobe bronchi can be considered normal, and the changes are particularly extensive in the posterior basilar segments of each lower lobe.

Bronchiectasis can be defined as dilatation of bronchi secondary to destruction of the muscular elements and elastic fibers in the bronchial walls caused by chronic infection. Collapse of these bronchial walls on expiration has been demonstrated by cinebronchography.

Although this patient had generalized bronchiectasis and was not a surgical candidate, some individuals develop a localized form involving a segment or a lobe, usually following infection. Posttuberculous bronchiectasis is a well-known entity, and a patient with this type of localized bronchiectasis may well benefit from surgery.

CASE D-8

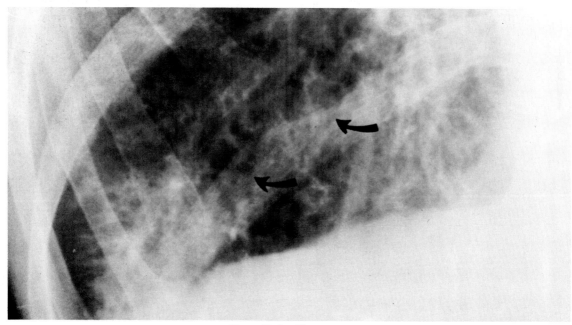

Figure D-8   Close-up

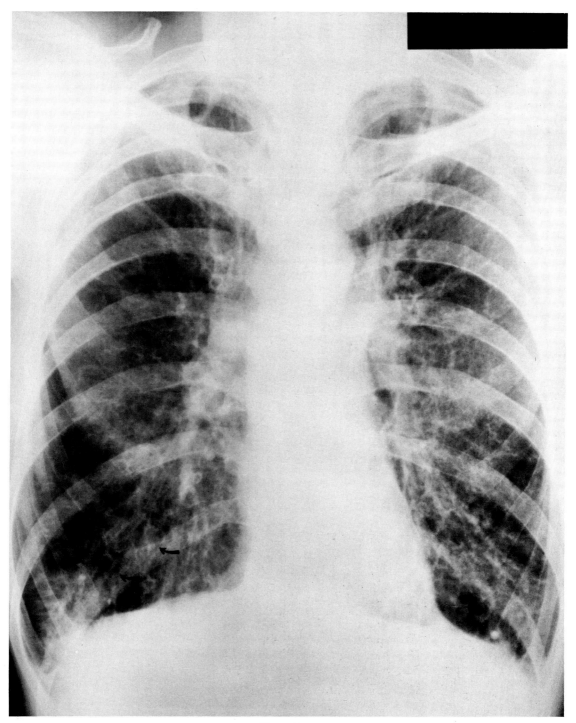

Figure D–8

Case D–8. This patient was a 60 year old white male who presented with a long history of a chronic productive cough and increasing dyspnea. How would you diagnose this patient's disease?

DISCUSSION, CASE D–8

While this patient's bronchiectasis is not nearly as obvious as that of the patient shown in Case D–7, this diagnosis can also be made on the basis of the plain radiograph of the chest. The curved arrows point to bronchiectatic changes in the right lower lobe, and close observation of the radiograph reveals multiple similar areas throughout both lungs. In patients with minimal bronchiectasis, the disease is often most obvious if they develop pneumonitis, because then the surrounding fluid-filled alveolar spaces cause the air-filled bronchiectatic bronchi to stand out. This patient is also obviously hyperaerated and has emphysema as well. The arrowhead once again points to a thickened, somewhat irregular bronchial wall secondary to chronic bronchitis.

CASE D–9

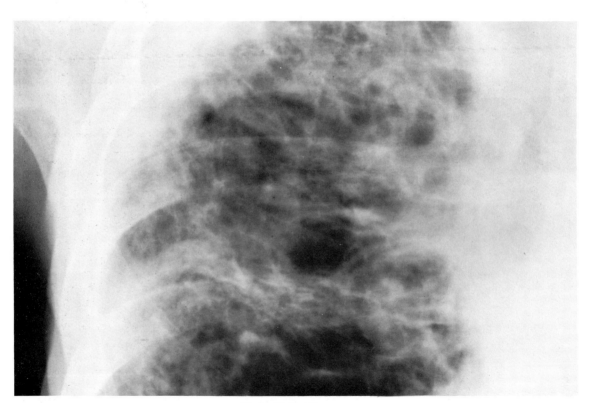

Figure D–9   Close-up

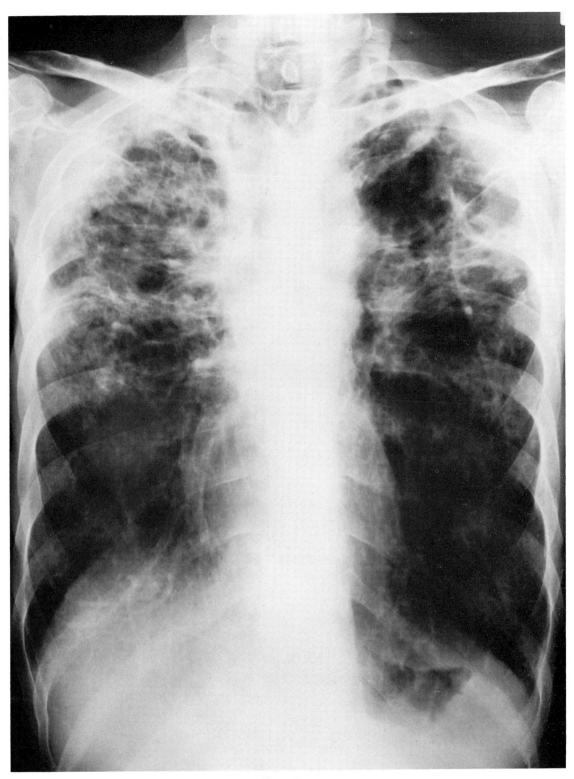

Figure D–9

Case D–9. This patient was a 56 year old white male who presented with increasing dyspnea and ankle edema. He had a 40 year history of chronic pulmonary disease with many recurrent episodes of pneumonitis. This was the first and only radiograph of this patient at our institution, and no previous radiographs were available for comparison. How would you report this case?

DISCUSSION, CASE D–9

This is a case of end-stage disease, and in essence this is all the radiologist can report. The patient has end-stage chronic obstructive airways disease as well as evidence of significant previous bilateral infection. Superimposed recent infection cannot be excluded.

At autopsy the patient was found to have severe bilateral upper lobe bronchiectasis, extensive interstitial fibrosis of the adjacent lung parenchyma, bronchopneumonia, bilateral severe necrotizing bronchitis, compensatory emphysema, and pulmonary arterial hypertension. There was no evidence that the patient had previous tuberculosis, histoplasmosis, or sarcoidosis.

In end-stage disease, however, one can never be certain that tuberculosis, histoplasmosis, or for that matter, any other infection is not present.

CASE D–10

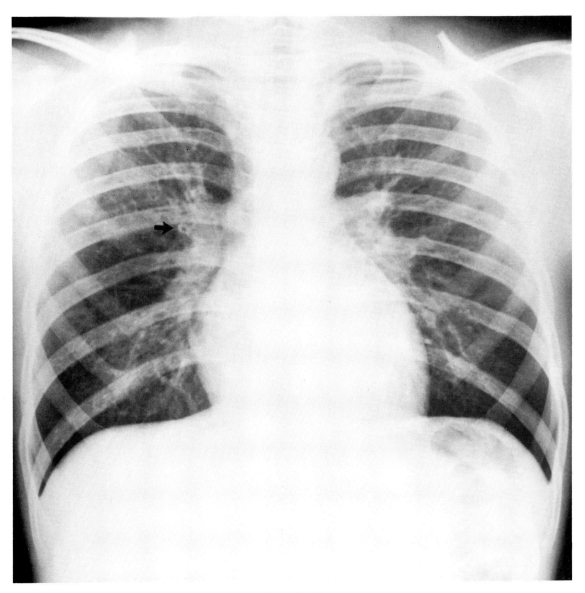

Figure D–10

Case D–10. This patient was a 7 year old white child who presented with an asthmatic attack.

CASE D-11 _____

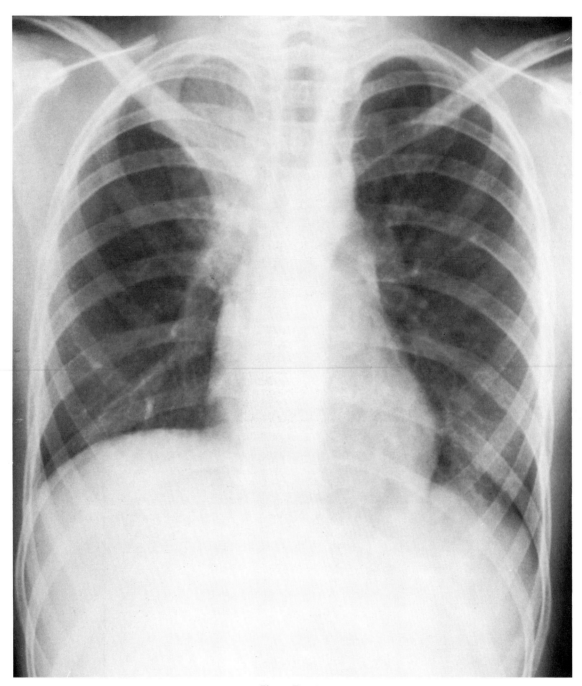

Figure D-11

Case D-11.   This patient was an 11 year old white child who presented with an asthmatic attack.

DISCUSSION, CASES D-10 and D-11

Figure D-10 presents the typical appearance of a child with an acute asthmatic attack. The hila are full, and there is thickening of the bronchial walls almost certainly caused by peribronchial edema. The edema demonstrated by the bronchus seen in cross section (arrowhead) undoubtedly plays a large role in making the hila appear full, and at times the vessels are somewhat blurred because of this edematous reaction. However, the hilar arteries are larger than normal, and this phenomenon deserves explanation as well. The peripheral asthmatic bronchospasm alters normal respiratory excursions and diminishes the effect of inspiration on peripheral arterial blood filling. Because the patient has difficulty in filling peripheral arteries, the hilar arteries are larger than normal.

Although the diagnosis is by no means proved, this child probably has exogenous asthma, that is, an antigen-antibody reaction secondary to an inhaled antigen. (This entity will be discussed again in Section E.)

Although the patient in Case D-11 presented in a very similar manner to the patient in Case D-10, the radiograph (Fig. D-11) shows other definitive changes. Did you note these changes? The radiograph demonstrates both a probable cause and a result of an acute attack of asthma. If you did not note these changes, go back and take another look at the radiograph before reading on.

The radiograph of this child shows two different processes, a pneumonitis along the left hemidiaphragm and atelectasis of the right upper lobe. The left lower lobe pneumonitis is almost certainly the cause of this patient's endogenous asthma, although this is not proved. The atelectasis in the right upper lobe, however, is the result of mucus that is plugging the right upper lobe bronchus, a rather common finding in patients with asthma.

The clinical presentation of pneumonitis in asthmatic patients is sometimes obvious, but frequently the presence of the pneumonitis is questionable. In addition, it is quite difficult to determine by auscultation whether the patient has an atelectatic segment or lobe. These two changes, pneumonitis and atelectasis, are therefore the major reasons, along with the possibility of pneumothorax, that clinicians request a roentgenographic examination of patients with asthma.

CASE D–12 _____

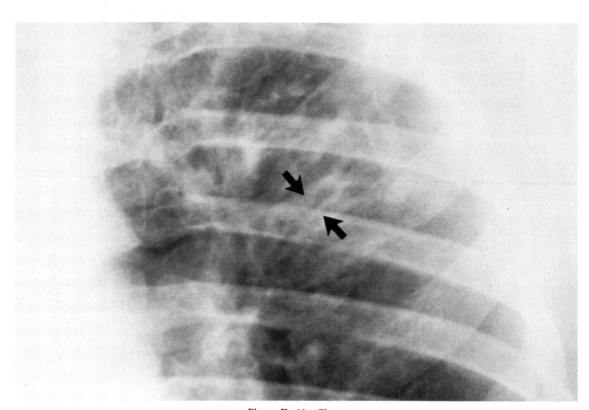

Figure D–12   Close-up

Figure D–12

Case D–12. This patient was a 26 year old white male who presented after many years of a chronic cough and increasing shortness of breath. The overall appearance of the chest and particularly the area outlined by arrows should enable you to make this diagnosis.

DISCUSSION, CASE D–12

Cystic fibrosis is the correct diagnosis. Don't let the age of the patient prevent you from making this diagnosis. There are significant numbers of patients with cystic fibrosis who initially present as adolescents or young adults and who live well into their middle years. It is in the diagnosis of these patients that the radiologist can play a major role. Some patients are not diagnosed earlier as having cystic fibrosis mostly because no one has thought of it. However, a hyperaerated chest, chronic pulmonary respiratory history, and thickened bronchial walls in any young patient should make one suspicious of cystic fibrosis.

As indicated previously, a number of acute and chronic diseases can cause thickening of the bronchial walls or peribronchial soft tissues. However, this observer has seen these thickened bronchial walls in the longitudinal plane (arrowhead) only in cystic fibrosis.

CASE D–13 _____

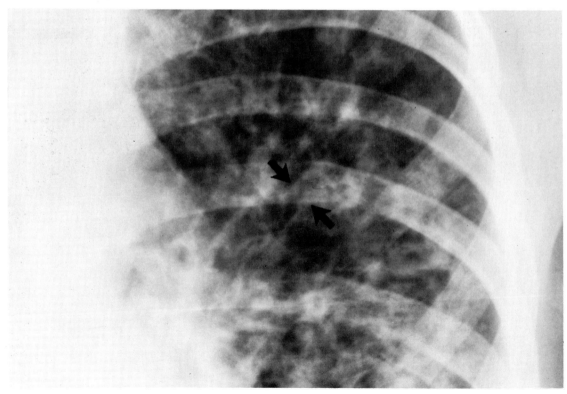

Figure D–13 Close-up

Figure D–13

Case D–13.   This patient was a 17 year old white female who presented with a long history of chronic respiratory disease, a chronic cough, and considerable increasing dyspnea.

DISCUSSION, CASE D–13

This is a much more advanced case of cystic fibrosis, as can be seen by the very extensive pulmonary parenchymal changes. The thickened bronchial walls are again obvious (arrowheads), but the patient also has multiple areas of chronic pneumonitis and atelectasis in the periphery as a result of the longstanding obstruction of the bronchi by thickened mucus secretions.

CASE D–14 _____

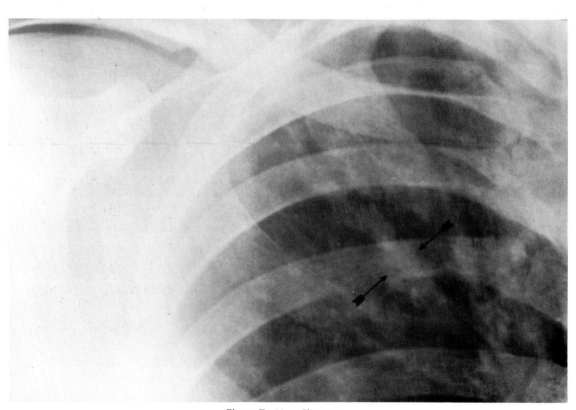

Figure D–14a   Close-up

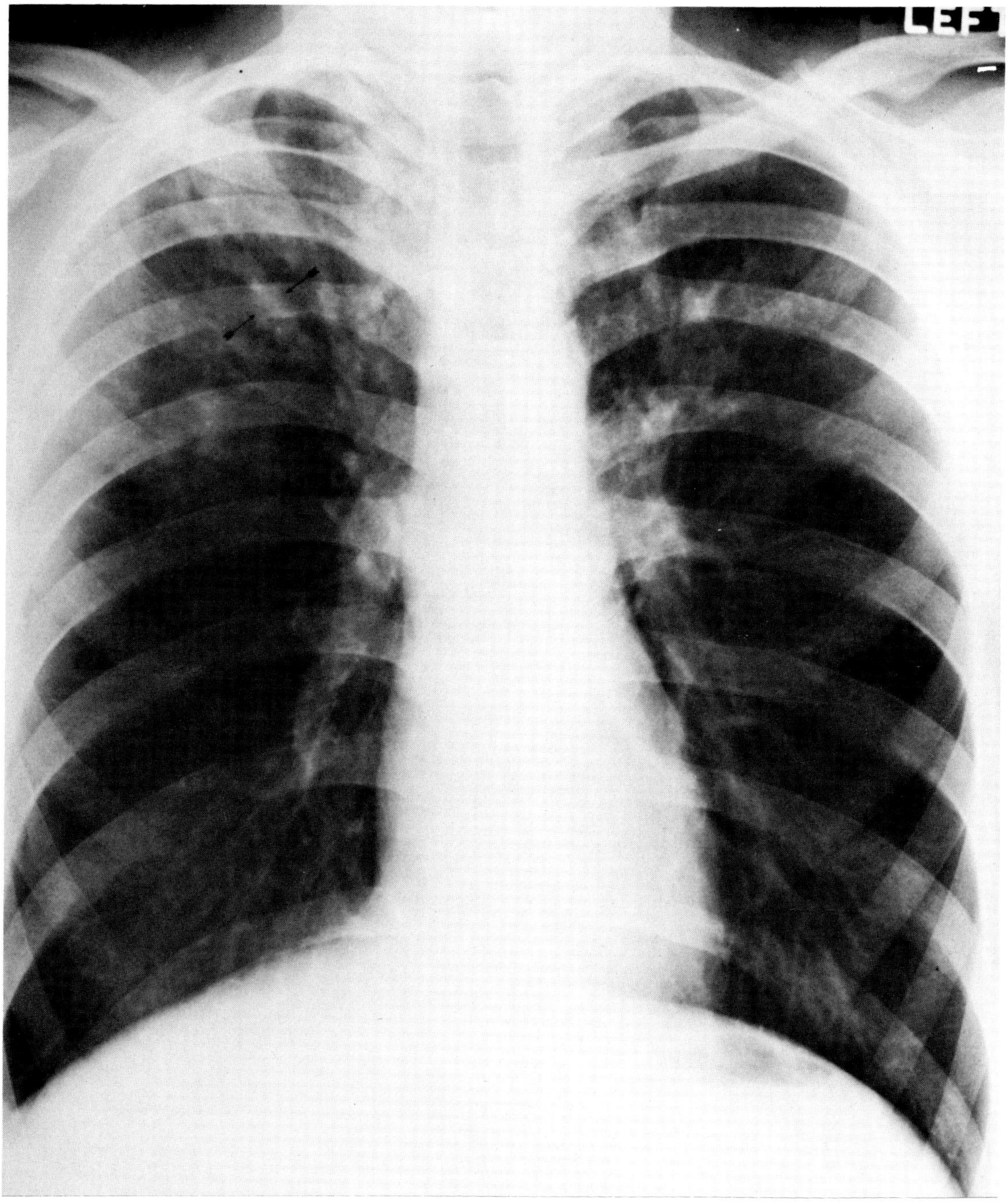

Figure D-14a

Case D-14a. This patient was an 18 year old white male who presented with a long history of asthmatic attacks, the last one of which was persistent enough to require hospitalization. What laboratory data would you request before making a conclusive diagnosis in this patient? Can you make the diagnosis without it? (A previous radiograph of the same patient (Fig. D-14b) is shown on the next page.)

CASE D–14 *CONTINUED*

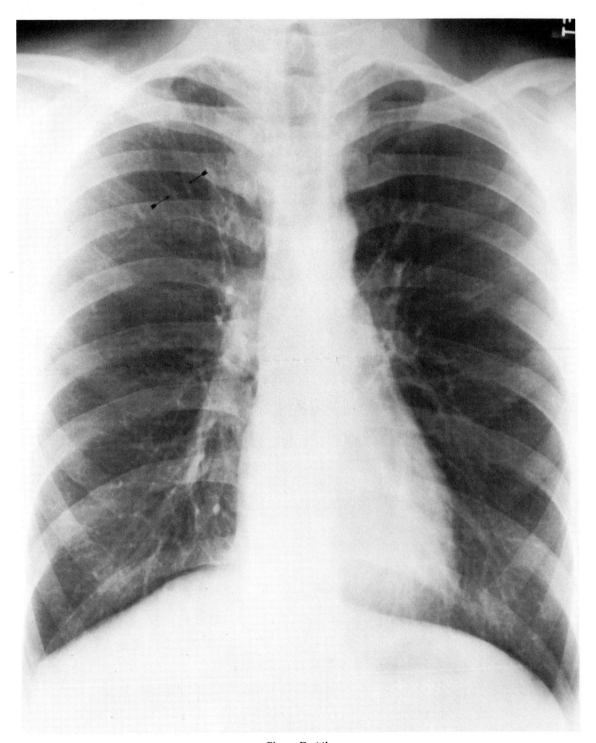

Figure D–14b

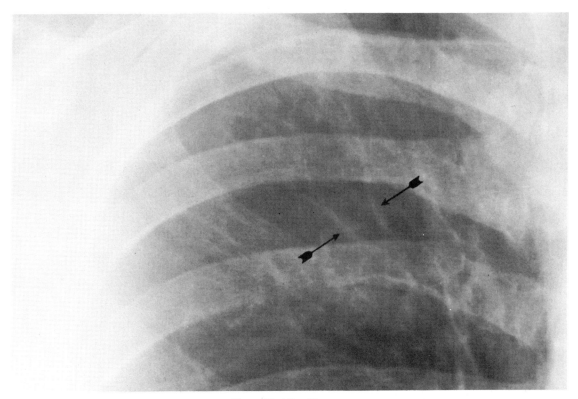

Figure D–14b   Close-up

Case D–14b. This radiograph of the same patient as shown in Figure D–14a was made 8 months earlier.

DISCUSSION, CASE D–14

The laboratory datum of marked interest in this patient is a blood eosinophilia of 24 per cent. Now you should definitely be able to make the diagnosis. Allergic aspergillosis is correct!

Aspergillus is a ubiquitous fungus, a complete discussion of which is outside the scope of this text. It attacks immunosuppressed patients in the form of pneumonitis, resides in the cysts and cavities formed by any number of other diseases, and has even been known to occur in otherwise normal individuals who have accidentally inhaled the fungus in massive amounts. Allergic aspergillosis, however, develops in asthmatics or in patients with cystic fibrosis. The fungus is found within the inspissated mucus in the bronchial tree. The typical radiographic appearance is dilatation of middle order bronchi that either are packed with the inspissated material containing the fungus as in Figure D–14a (arrows) or are empty and air-filled as demonstrated in Figure D–14b (arrows).

CASE D-15 _____

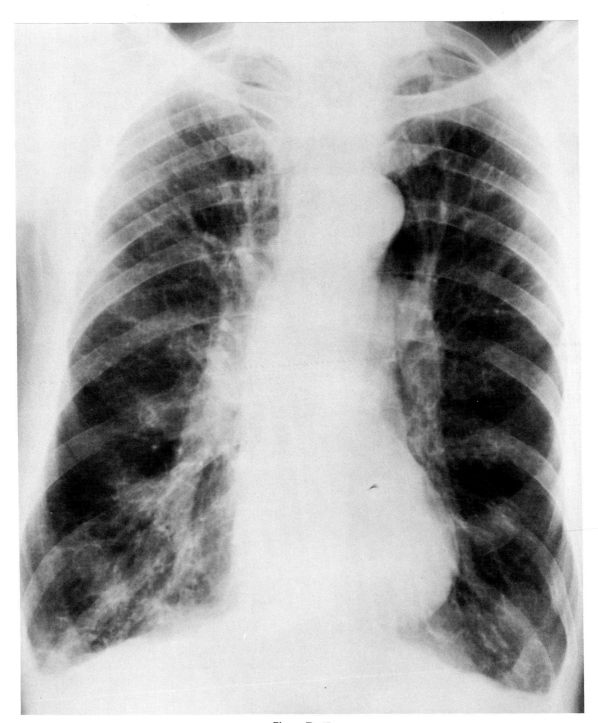

Figure D–15a

Case D–15a.   This patient was a 75 year old white male who had been chronically short of breath for many years and who presented to the emergency suite with acute dyspnea. What is your diagnosis? (A previous radiograph of this patient [Fig. D–15b] is shown on the next page.)

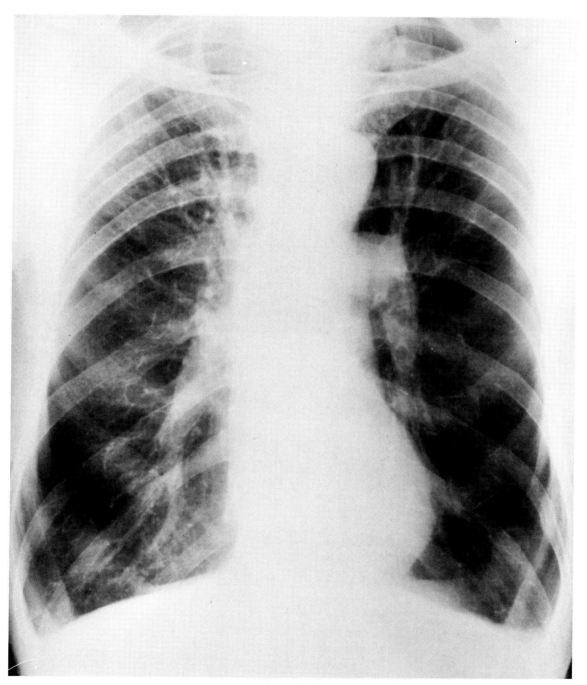

Figure D–15b

Case D–15b. This radiograph was made several years before of the same patient as shown in Figure D–15a.

DISCUSSION, CASE D–15

The correct diagnosis is congestive heart failure. Acute cardiac decompensation and pulmonary edema in a patient with obstructive airways disease is difficult to recognize but should always be suspected under the circumstances just noted. The patient's pulmonary vascular bed is so poor that he can demonstrate pulmonary edema only in his lower lobes, and the edema is best seen on the right side. If you claim that pneumonitis cannot be excluded radiographically, you are correct. Communication with the patient's physician, however, should clarify the diagnosis without much difficulty. There will be times, however, when a patient will present with pneumonitis and cardiac decompensation, and under such circumstances it is virtually impossible to tell whether the new disease is due to pneumonitis, pulmonary edema, or both. This patient's heart, however, is considerably larger than expected for his emphysematous chest.

REFERENCES

1. Burrows, B., Fletcher, C. M., Heard, B. E., et al.: The emphysematous and bronchial types of chronic airways obstruction. Lancet, 1:830–835, 1966.
2. Burrows, B., Niden, A. H., Fletcher, C. M., et al.: Clinical types of chronic obstructive lung disease in London and in Chicago. Am. Rev. Resp. Dis., 90:14–27, 1964.
3. Chan-Yeung, M., Chase, W. H., Trapp, W., et al.: Allergic bronchopulmonary aspergillosis. Chest, 59(1):33–39, 1971.
4. Feist, J.: Selective cinebronchography in obstructive and restrictive pulmonary disease. Am. J. Roentgenol., 99:543–554, 1967.
5. Filley, G. F.: Emphysema and chronic bronchitis: clinical manifestations and their physiologic significance. Med. Clin. North Am., 51:283–292, 1967.
6. Fraser, R.: The radiologist and obstructive airway disease. Am. J. Roentgenol., 120:737–775, 1974.
7. Freundlich, I. M., and Dure-Smith, P.: Aspiration bronchography: a new look at a simple non-instrumental technique. J. Can. Assoc. Radiol., 22:201–205, 1971.
8. Hogg, J. C., Macklem, P. T., and Thurlbeck, W. M.: Site and nature of airway obstruction in chronic obstructive lung disease. N. Engl. J. Med., 278:1355–1360, 1968.
9. Milne, E., and Bass, H.: Roentgenologic diagnosis of early chronic obstructive pulmonary disease. J. Can. Assoc. Radiol., 20:3–15, 1969.
10. Morse, J. O., Lebowitz, M. D., Knudson, R. J., et al.: Relation of protease inhibitor phenotypes to obstructive lung diseases in a community. N. Engl. J. Med., 296:1190–1194, 1977.
11. Simon, G.: The plain radiograph in relation to lung physiology. Radiol. Clin. North Am., 11(1):3–16, 1973.
12. Simon, M., Sasahara, A. A., and Cannilla, J. E.: The radiology of pulmonary hypertension. Semin. Roentgenol., 2(1):368–388, 1967.
13. Wood, R. E., Boat, T. F., and Doershuk, C. F.: Cystic fibrosis. In Murray, J. F. (ed.): Lung Disease — State of the Art 1975–1976. New York, American Lung Association, 1977, pp. 275–320.
14. Zimmerman, R. A., and Miller, W. T.: Pulmonary aspergillosis. Am. J. Roentgenol., 109:505–515, 1970.

If the answers to the four questions asked in Sections A, B, C, and D are all no, then we are left with a diffuse pulmonary disease in a patient who is not known to be immunosuppressed. The disease is predominantly interstitial but not grossly nodular. It may be granular, reticular, mottled, or linear, and any hyperaeration present is secondary.

Decision 1. Once again the decision 1 must be whether interstitial pulmonary edema is present. One can never assume that interstitial changes are old or chronic without having previous radiographs for comparison, and such an assumption on the part of the radiologist might actually lead to a delay in the proper management of a patient with acute pulmonary edema.

Decision 2. The second decision should be the possibility of an acute, widespread viral pneumonitis, which may demonstrate a diffuse, predominantly interstitial pattern not unlike that of interstitial pulmonary edema. Fortunately, this presentation is rare except in influenza epidemics, as these patients are desperately ill. In such patients, the lung's inability to maintain a satisfactory gas exchange forces the use of a high percentage of oxygen in therapy, and this can then lead to the adult respiratory distress syndrome.

Decision 3. If the first two decisions of this section are answered negatively, then we move to Decision 3, which involves hypersensitivity reactions. Type I, type II, and type III immune reactions will be considered.

TYPE I IMMUNE REACTION. In this type of immune reaction, IgE is bound to tissue mast cells, which elaborate histamines and other products when the antibody IgE combines with the allergen. The immediate skin test is positive, and two examples of type I reactions follow:

1. extrinsic asthma
2. anaphylactic reaction

An immediate hypersensitivity reaction to any drug, for example, intravenous contrast material, may produce a diffuse reaction in the lungs. The type of immediate reaction depends upon which system is affected, as follows:

a. skin: urticaria
b. gastrointestional system: nausea and vomiting
c. respiratory system: laryngospasm, bronchospasm, and acute hypersensitivity pneumonitis.
d. vascular system: hypotension.

One must next know whether the patient has hemoptysis or hematuria. These clinical signs suggest a type II immune reaction.

TYPE II IMMUNE REACTION. In a type II immune reaction, the antibodies present are IgG- and IgM-dependent, cytotoxic, and tissue-specific. Other classes of antibodies as well as the complement system are involved. This type of reaction is also known as basement membrane disease. The alveolar and glomerular basement membranes are altered, possibly by a virus. This altered membrane then combines with the antibody. Pulmonary hemorrhage is the common finding in this type of reaction. Some examples of a type II reaction are

a. Goodpasture's syndrome
b. hemolytic anemia, leukopenia, and thrombocytopenia purpura
c. primary hemosiderosis (?)

TYPE III IMMUNE REACTION. Historical information is once again necessary in order for us to consider a type III immune reaction. The radiologist must know whether the patient has a history of inhalation of any toxic industrial particles or any known antigen. In addition, a type III immune reaction that is observed in the lungs may be caused by a known collagen vascular disease.

The type III immune reaction is predominantly IgG- and IgM-dependent. However, all classes of antibodies and the complement system are involved. It is also known as immune-complex disease (Arthus reaction). Immune-complex disease produces interstitial pneumonitis with vasculitis and often granulomatosis. It has also been called hypersensitivity angiitis, allergic angiitis, and allergic alveolitis. Allergic alveolitis is probably the best descriptive term, as both vasculitis and granulomata occur only variably with immune-complex reactions. Examples of a type III reaction may be broken into the following two types: (a) airborne or extrinsic allergic alveolitis and (b) bloodborne or intrinsic allergic alveolitis. The list of antigens which may cause extrinsic allergic alveolitis continues to grow, and only some of the conditions caused by those antigens are included in the following list:

a. farmer's lung
b. mushroom worker's disease
c. sequoiosis
d. bagassosis
e. maple bark disease
f. pigeon breeder's lung
g. byssinosis

(*Note:* Asbestosis, and berylliosis can also be included in the extrinsic allergic alveolitis group.) Bloodborne or intrinsic allergic alveolitis is a pulmonary reaction to a systemic autoimmune process. Some of the diseases which belong in this group are the following:

a. progressive systemic sclerosis
b. rheumatoid arthritis
c. lupus erythematosus
d. polyarthritis nodosa
e. Wegener's granulomatosis
f. Sjögren's syndrome
g. Polymyositis and dermatomyositis

Other type III reactions are generally considered to be idiopathic:

a. pulmonary infiltrates with eosinophilia (PIE syndrome)
b. tropical eosinophilic pneumonitis
c. idiosyncratic drug reaction

Chronic eosinophilic pneumonitis, also called pulmonary infiltrates with eosinophilia syndrome, is undoubtedly a hypersensitivity reaction, but it is one in which the antigen cannot be identified. The pneumonitis is frequently peripheral, at times with an extensive alveolar component. The clear central portion of the lungs characteristic of this entity has suggested to some observers that it is the opposite of the usual radiographic picture of central and symmetric pulmonary edema.

The breakdown of pulmonary immunologic diseases into the various types is often not clear-cut. A drug reaction, for example, may be due to a type I and a type III response, while Goodpasture's pulmonary-renal syndrome is probably type II and III reactions combined. If granulomata are present in any immunologic event, then a type IV, T-cell mediated reaction has also occurred.

Decision 4. Decision 4 involves a number of rare entities known collectively as the lymphoproliferative disorders. In the rapidly advancing field of immunology, however, these diseases, along with multiple myeloma, are also called plasma cell dyscrasias. The plasma cell is derived from the B-cell lymphocyte and is responsible for the production of most of the immunoglobulins (antibodies). Some of the disorders in this fascinating and poorly understood group of diseases are related to the plasma cell itself (as in multiple myeloma), some are probably related to a cell that is intermediate between the B cell and the plasma cell (as in Waldenström's macroglobulinemia), and the heavy-chain disorders seem to be dyscrasias of the B-cell lymphocyte itself. Like multiple myeloma, plasma cell leukemia, and lymphocytic leukemia, the entities that follow are all related to malignancies of the plasma cell or of its B cell precursor:

a. primary macroglobulinemia (Waldenström's disease)
b. heavy-chain disease
c. amyloidosis
d. pseudolymphoma

The pulmonary parenchymal changes seen in the diseases just listed are related for the most part to interstitial cellular infiltrations and to a lesser degree to the deposition of abnormal immunoglobulins. Amyloidosis is also related to the plasma cell dyscrasias, and it is likely that some of the parenchymal change seen in this group of diseases is caused by the deposition of amyloid as well.

Decision 5. Decision 5 involves diseases that are at least partially fibrotic and fit in no other category. The diagnosis is almost always made by lung biopsy, except when asbestosis is obvious.

a. asbestosis (almost always with pleural thickening)
b. usual interstitial pneumonia (UIP) — possibly a type III response
c. desquamative interstitial pneumonia (DIP)
d. lymphocytic interstitial pneumonia (LIP) — possibly one of the lymphoproliferative disorders.
e. giant cell interstitial pneumonia (GIP)

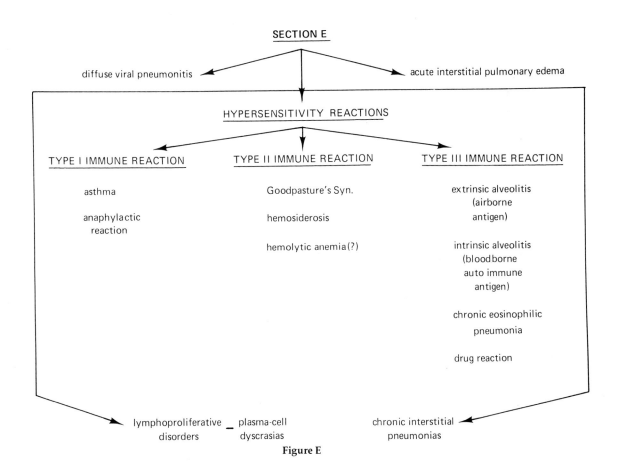

Figure E

CASE E-1

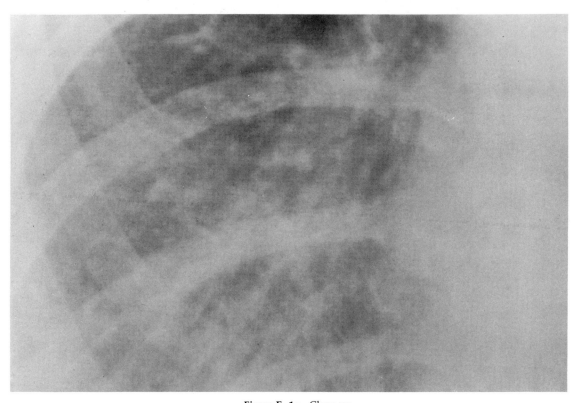

Figure E–1a   Close-up

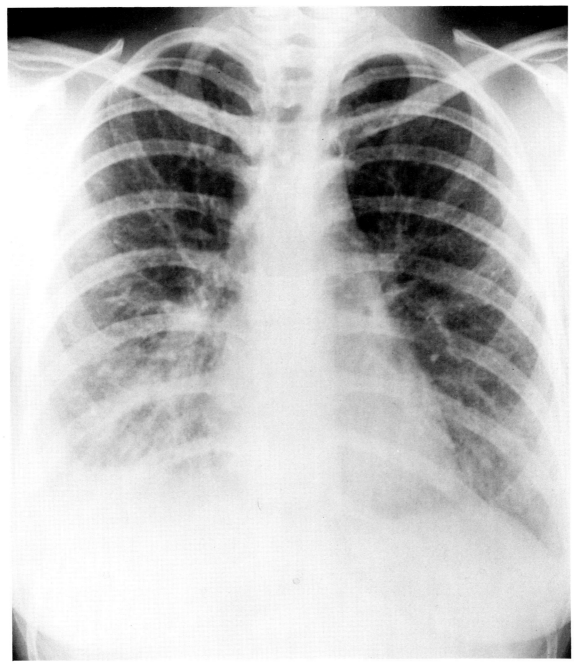

Figure E–1a

Case E–1a. This patient was a 21 year old white female hair stylist who presented in the emergency suite with dyspnea, fever, chills, and burning chest pain. These symptoms were preceded by a week of myalgia, pharyngitis, and diarrhea. The patient had been entirely well previously, except for episodic secondary amenorrhea for which she had been placed on birth control pills. Figure E–1a was made on the day of admission and Figure E–1b on the sixth hospital day. What do you think of this patient's diffuse chest disease? Compare this case with the following one (Case E–2). Cases E–1 and E–2 are discussed as a unit after Case E–2.

CASE E–1 *CONTINUED*

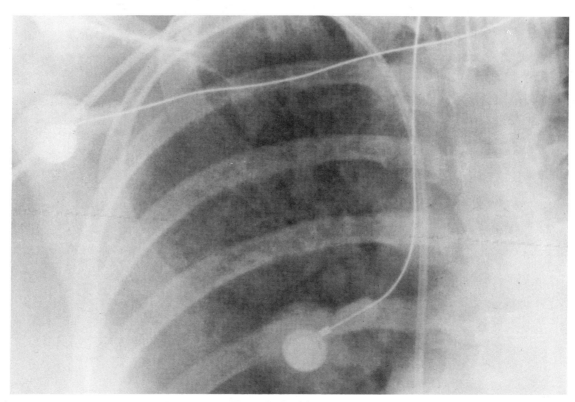

Figure E–1b   Close-up

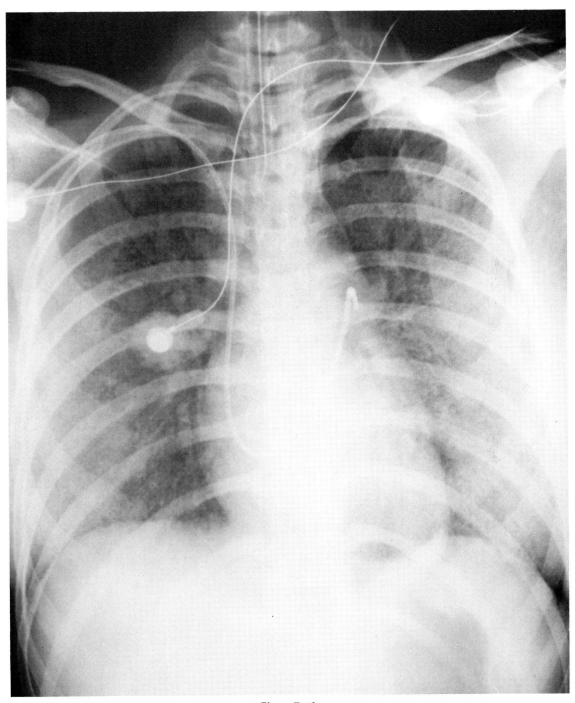

Figure E-1b

Case E-1b. This radiograph of the same patient shown in Figure E-1a was made on the sixth hospital day. The patient's condition had deteriorated, with an obvious diffusion impairment and a low arterial oxygen saturation. What do you think is the cause of this patient's diffuse disease?

CASE E–2

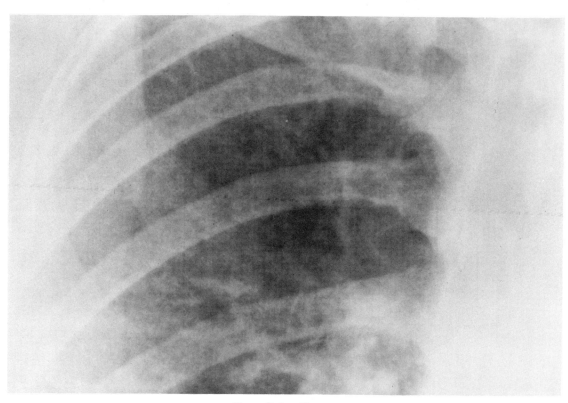

Figure E–2a   Close-up

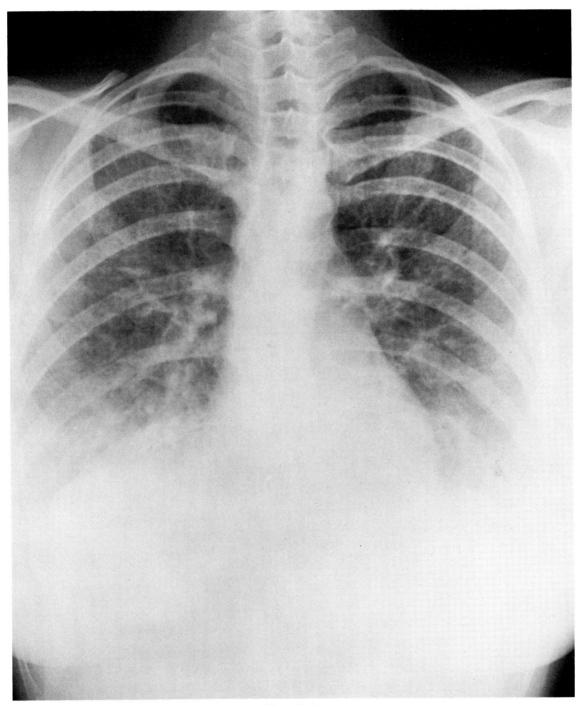

Figure E-2a

Case E-2a. This patient was a 22 year old white female college student who presented in the emergency suite with acute dyspnea, pleuritic chest pain, fever, and a nonproductive cough. She had been recently treated for this illness with penicillin, which was not effective. There was no significant past history. Obviously, the two young female patients in this case and the preceding one had similar illnesses. What is your diagnosis? Additional radiographs of this patient are seen on the next two pages.

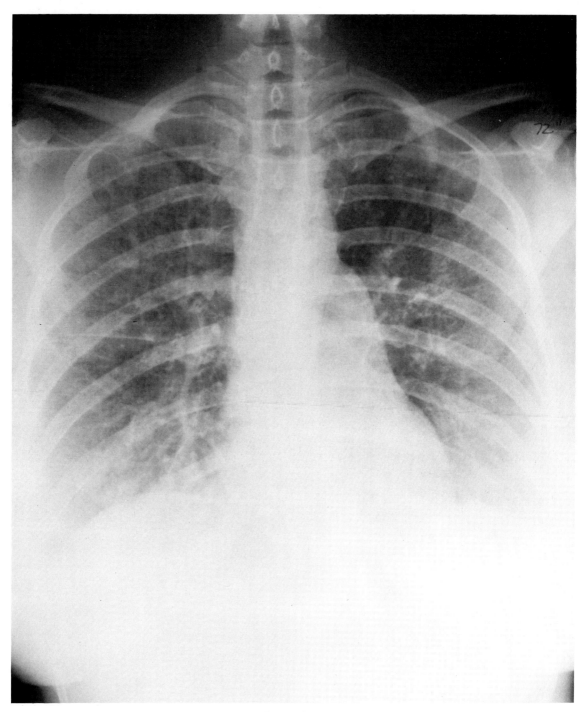

Figure E–2b

Case E–2b. This radiograph of the same patient shown in Figure E–2a was made 3 days later.

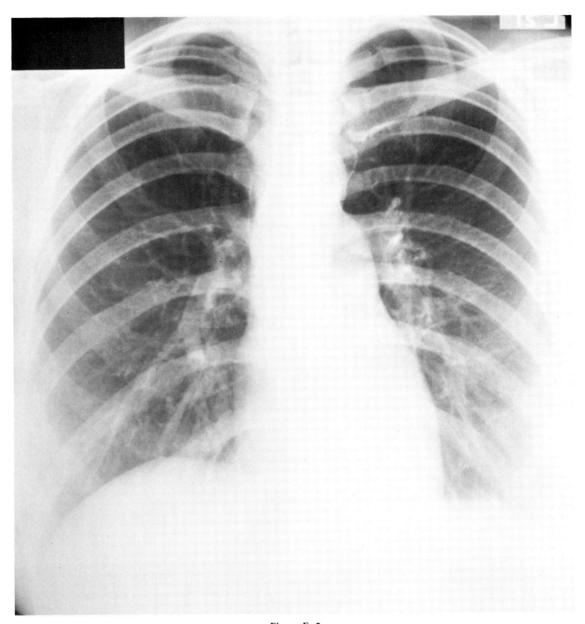

Figure E-2c

Case E-2c. This radiograph of the same patient shown in Figures E-2a and E-2b was made several months after her discharge from the hospital.

DISCUSSION, CASES E–1 and E–2

The patients in these two cases are similar in that both had diffuse viral pneumonitis. The patient demonstrated in Figure E–1a died of her illness on the twenty-second hospital day. At autopsy a diffuse interstitial pneumonitis was found, which had previously been proved to be caused by influenza B. There were, in addition, pneumothoraces and multiple areas of bronchial pneumonia and organizing pneumonitis secondary to superimposed bacterial infection. Multiple small pulmonary thromboemboli were also present. This patient's demise was secondary to many factors, but the underlying and primary cause was the diffuse interstitial influenza pneumonitis. The interstitial inflammatory changes just described were aggravated by the superimposed adult respiratory distress syndrome secondary to the oxygen therapy, which was necessary throughout the patient's hospital course to sustain her life. The pneumothoraces, subsequent pulmonary collapse, and superimposed bacterial infection also played a significant role in this patient's demise. The questionable history of inhalation of hair spray was not thought to be of any clinical importance nor was the history of taking birth control pills, despite the evidence of pulmonary thromboemboli found at the post-mortem.

The patient shown in Figure D–2a was discharged on the fifth hospital day and made an uneventful recovery. Although clinically there was no question that she had a diffuse viral pneumonitis, a specific virus was never isolated.

The radiologic similarity of these two cases in their early stages is striking, and at the time of admission it was certainly not possible to predict the eventual outcome. One can only speculate about the differences between these two patients, and it is probable that the pathogenicity of the viral organism was the most significant factor. In general, however, immune mechanisms play a significant role in the host response to a diffuse viral illness.

The most important role for the radiologist in this type of case is to alert the clinician to the widespread nature of the parenchymal interstitial disease, so that all appropriate supportive measures can be promptly initiated. It is indeed fortunate that viral pneumonitis is most often a local process and is well handled by host defense mechanisms. The patient shown in Figure E–1a, however, brings home to the radiologist the fear that is induced in epidemiologic circles by the possibility of an influenza pandemic.

CASE E-3 _____

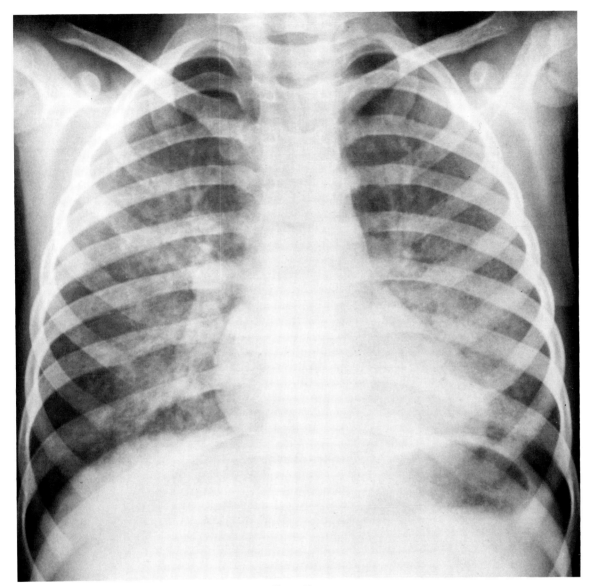

Figure E-3a

Case E-3a.   This patient was a 5 year old white male child who present-ed with hemoptysis and dyspnea on exertion. He had had at least two other similar episodes, the first of which had occurred approximately 2 years be-fore this admission. What is your differential diagnosis of this child's dis-ease?

The next two radiographs are of the same patient.

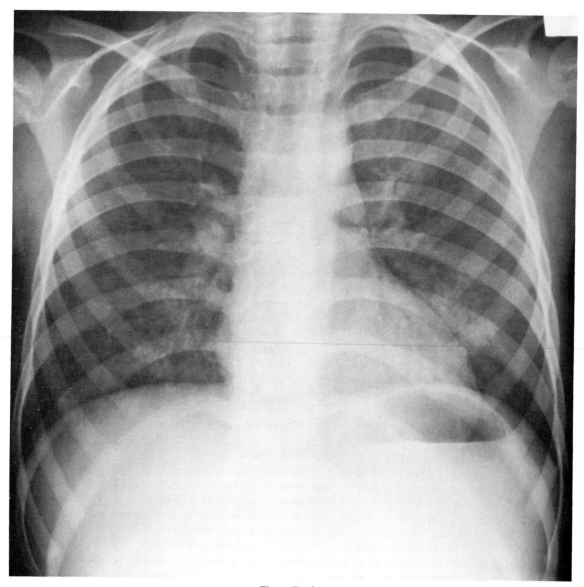

Figure E–3b

Case E–3b. This radiograph of the same child shown in Figure E–3a was made 4 weeks later. Several urinalyses and the peripheral blood count and smear were normal except for slight anemia. Can you now make the diagnosis?

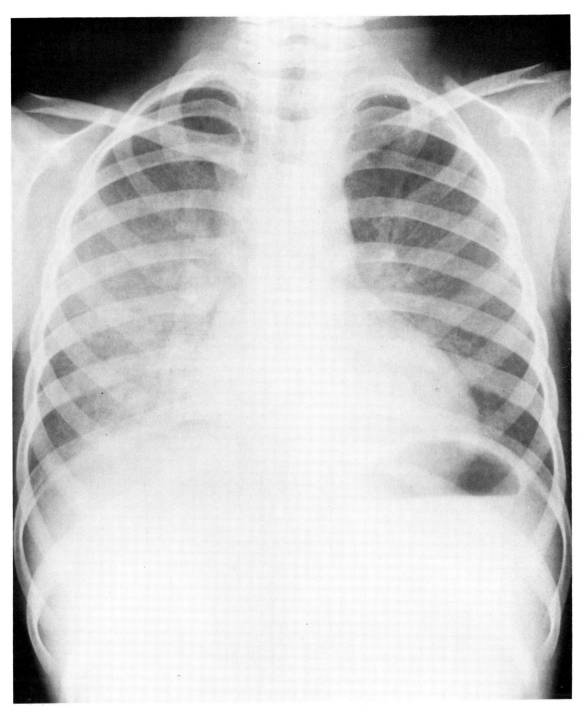

Figure E–3c

Case E–3c. This is a radiograph of the same child made 2 weeks after the radiograph seen in Figure E–3b.

DISCUSSION, CASE E–3

In a child with hemoptysis, several possible causes of the disorder must be considered. One that must be given initial consideration is the possibility that blood is being aspirated from a bleeding site in the upper respiratory tract. However, this possibility is usually rapidly excluded by direct visualization of the nasopharynx and oropharynx. Otherwise, in children with no cardiovascular illness there are three primary considerations — Goodpasture's syndrome, leukemia, and idiopathic primary hemosiderosis. It has been noted previously that leukemic children with diminished platelets or thrombocytopenia can bleed into their lungs. The peripheral blood count or an examination of the bone marrow will determine whether the patient has leukemia. If the urinalysis is normal, Goodpasture's syndrome can usually be excluded, although in some cases renal biopsy is necessary. The correct diagnosis in Case E–3, therefore, is idiopathic hemosiderosis. Evidence of the waxing and waning of the pulmonary infiltrates secondary to the hemorrhage is clearly seen in Figures E–3b and E–3c. The diagnosis is usually established when macrophages containing significant amounts of hemosiderin are found in the sputum or in gastric aspirates. Occasionally a lung biopsy is necessary to make the diagnosis.

Normal pulmonary tissue absorbs blood fairly rapidly. Even in this child, who clearly has a poorly understood abnormality of his alveolocapillary membrane, the blood was cleared from his lungs. In those patients who acquire the adult respiratory distress syndrome, however, the blood products cannot be cleared from their lungs because of extensive destruction of the alveolocapillary membrane and damage to the surfactant system.

This child represents a particularly fascinating case of an unusual disease. He has three male siblings, in one of whom the same diagnosis has been proved, and in a second of whom it is suspected. Of course, this leads one to suspect a congenital etiology in this idiopathic illness, but the occurrence of the same disease in siblings can also be explained by a transmittable infection. If this disease is also a type II immune response and similar in that regard to Goodpasture's syndrome, then alteration of the alveolocapillary membrane by a virus cannot be excluded as a possible etiology.

CASE E-4 _____

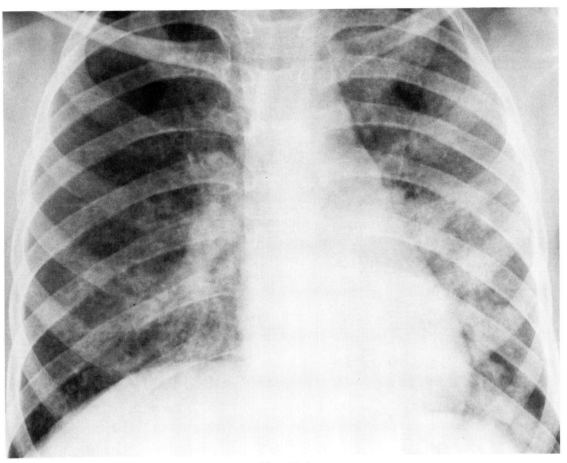

Figure E-4

Case E-4.   This patient was an 8 year old white female who presented after 5 months of a cough that began with an upper respiratory infection. The cough had been nonproductive, and there was no hemoptysis, but occasional vomiting with hematemesis was reported. The peripheral blood count and smear were normal except for moderate anemia. Additional laboratory data revealed proteinuria and elevated BUN and serum creatine levels. What is your diagnosis in this case?

DISCUSSION, CASE E–4

Despite the absence of hemoptysis, the radiograph and laboratory data alone point toward Goodpasture's syndrome as the most probable diagnosis. In this child, renal and pulmonary biopsy were carried out, both of which confirmed the diagnosis.

Goodpasture's syndrome is thought to be a type II immune response, probably combined with a type III, with specific involvement of the basement membrane of the glomeruli, leading to chronic glomerulonephritis. These changes were evident in the renal biopsy performed on the child presented in Figure E–4, and the lung biopsy revealed old as well as recent pulmonary hemorrhage.

CASE E–5

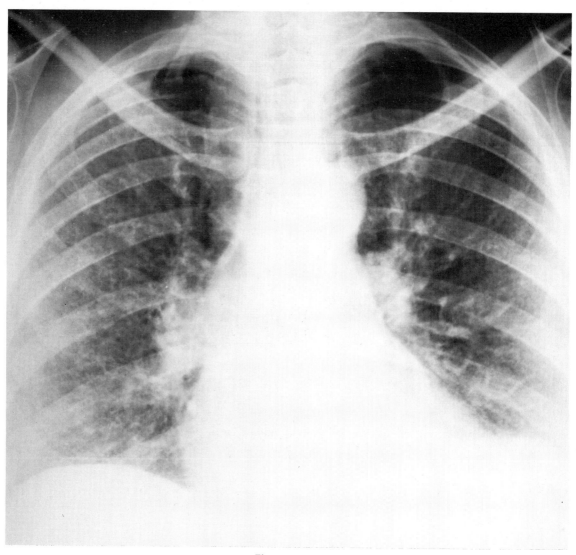

Figure E–5a

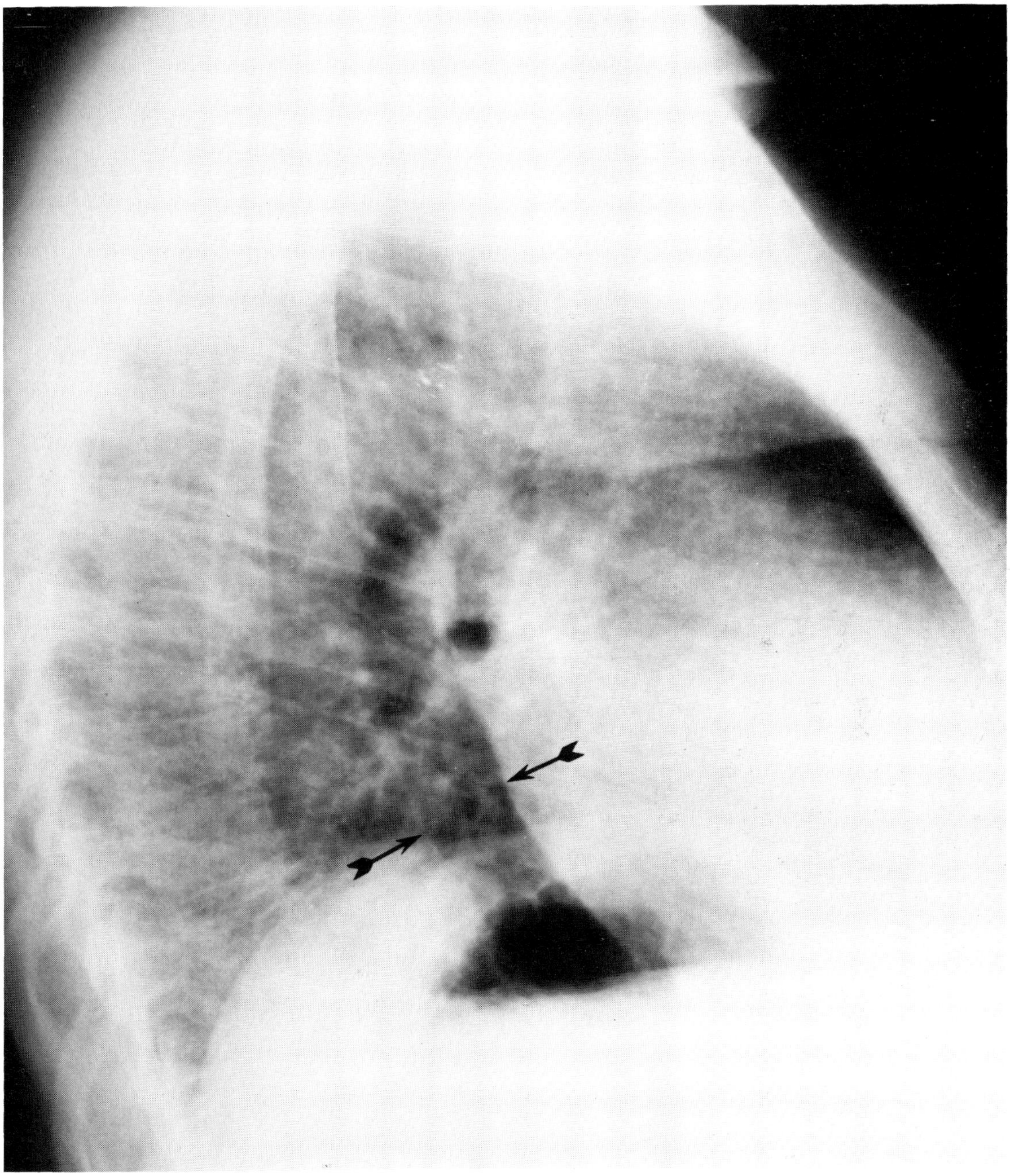

Figure E-5b

Case E-5.   This patient is a 48 year old white female with a known chronic disease (Figs. E-5a and E-5b). What is your diagnosis in this case?

DISCUSSION, CASE E–5

The arrows in the radiograph outline a moderately distended, air-filled esophagus. This finding, in addition to the minor interstitial thickening seen in each lower lobe, should allow you to make the diagnosis without further clinical information. If your answer is progressive systemic sclerosis, you are absolutely right.

This entity is, of course, one of the collagen vascular diseases in which the antigen-antibody complex is bloodborne; this is another way of saying that it is an autoimmune disease. The majority of patients with progressive systemic sclerosis present initially with dermal or gastrointestinal symptomatology, and chest manifestations usually appear at a later stage. In this particular case, however, the diagnosis can be made from the chest radiograph alone by noting the basilar interstitial fibrosis and the distended, air-filled esophagus.

CASE E–6

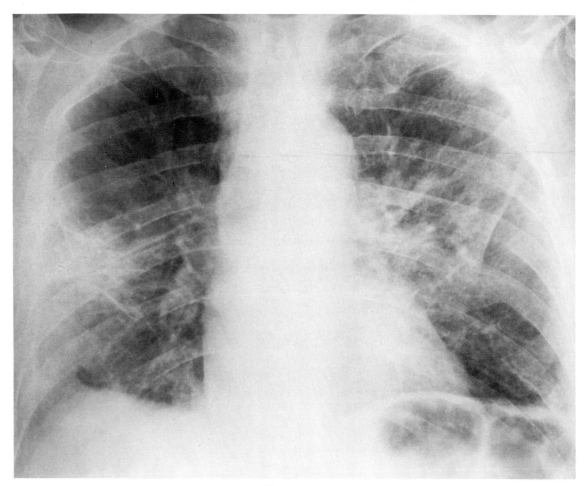

Figure E–6a

Case E–6a. This patient was a 58 year old white male who presented with increasing dyspnea and intermittent pleuritic chest pain. He had been followed for a number of years for a known chronic disease. What chronic disease do you think he had, and how would you describe the chest manifestations of that disease?

The radiograph on the next page is of the same patient.

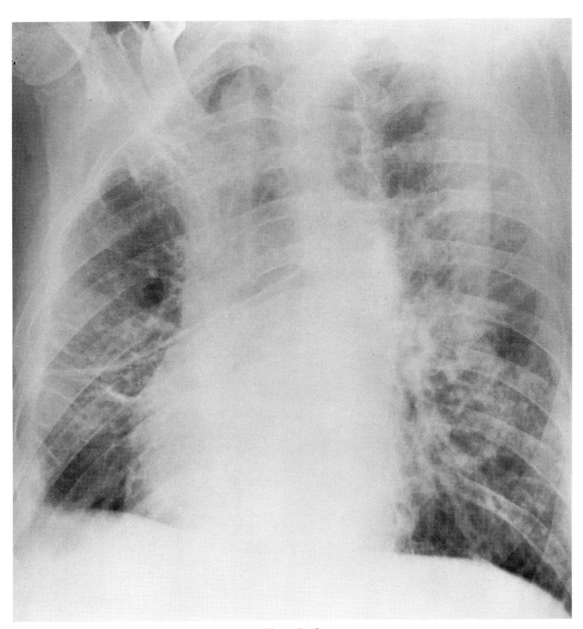

Figure E–6b

Case E–6b. This oblique radiograph of the same patient shown in Figure E–6a was made several weeks later, at which time he still had right pleuritic chest pain as well as dyspnea on exertion.

DISCUSSION, CASE E–6

If you diagnosed the chronic disease as one belonging to the collagen vascular group, you are correct. The patient had suffered from known rheumatoid arthritis for several years, and the radiographs demonstrate the two most common manifestations of rheumatoid lung — pleuritis with effusion and parenchymal fibrosis. The radiographs show considerable fibrosis, mostly in the lower lobes, as well as a small pleural effusion. The high position of the diaphragm is almost certainly secondary to the interstitial fibrosis, which has resulted in a restrictive pulmonary disease.

The great majority of patients who develop pulmonary parenchymal or pleural changes have had well established rheumatoid arthritis for varying periods of time. It is rare to see the chest manifestations of rheumatoid arthritis before the diagnosis has been established.

Each of the collagen vascular diseases can affect the lungs, but progressive systemic sclerosis and rheumatoid arthritis are by far the most common. Patients with lupus erythematosus may present with panserositis, that is, pleuritis and pericarditis, almost always with effusions. These changes in the chest are at times accompanied by pneumonitis. However, it may be quite difficult to determine whether the pleural, pericardial, and parenchymal changes are caused by chronic renal failure or by the primary disease. The pulmonary radiographic manifestations of polyarteritis nodosa and Sjögren's syndrome are rare, and Wegener's granulomatosis has already been discussed in Section B.

Ankylosing spondylitis is not usually included in the collagen vascular group of diseases, but uncommonly, this entity may also produce pulmonary parenchymal fibrosis in the upper lobes.

CASE E-7

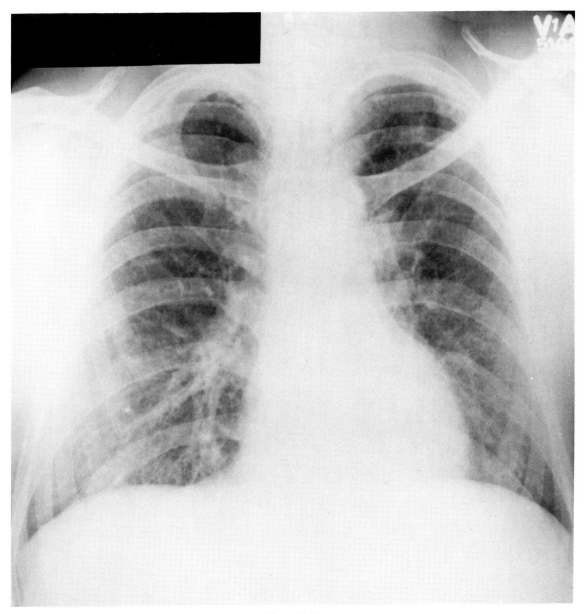

Figure E-7a

Case E-7a. This patient was a 56 year old white male who presented with a 12 year history of intermittent wheezing and dyspnea. Laboratory data was not helpful. What is your differential diagnosis? Additional radiographs of this patient are demonstrated on the next two pages.

CASE E–7 *CONTINUED*

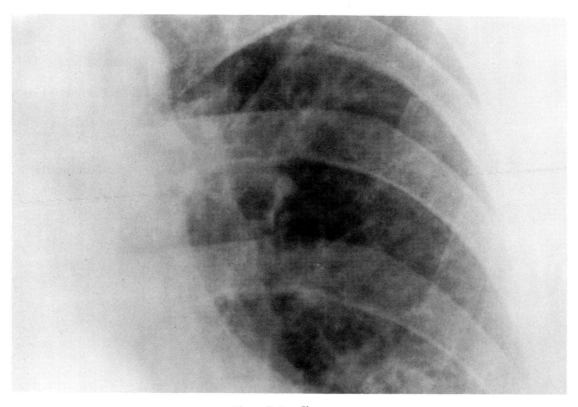

Figure E–7a Close-up

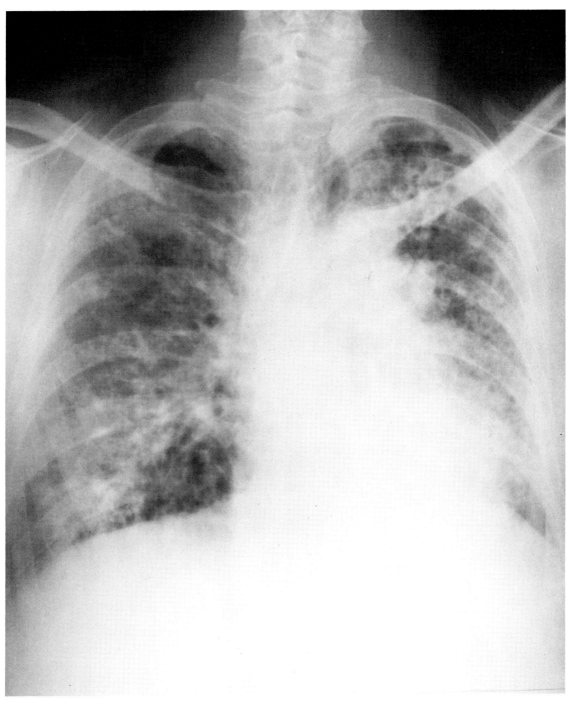

Figure E-7b

Case E-7b. This is a radiograph of the patient in Figure E-7a made 10 years later.

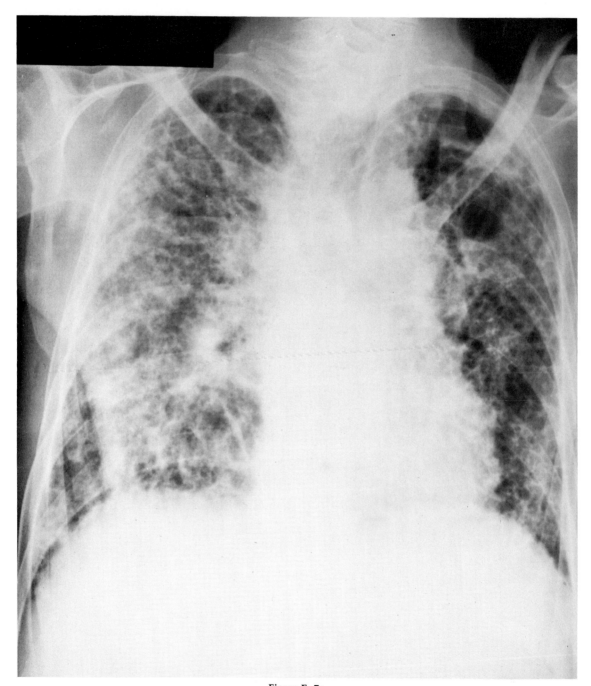

Figure E–7c

Case E–7c. This radiograph of the same patient shown in Figures E–7a and, E–7b was made approximately 6 years after the radiograph in Figure E–7b and 16 years after the original one.

DISCUSSION, CASE E–7

In analyzing the initial radiograph we find minimal interstitial changes, mostly in a central position and somewhat more marked on the left side. Let us use this case as a model and follow the diagnostic schema from its beginning in Section A through to this point in Section E. The patient is not immuno-suppressed, has no known neoplasm, and is not taking medication. He certainly does not have a nodular disease, airspace filling, or evidence of significant hyperaeration or pulmonary arterial hypertension. Therefore, this case must be considered within Section E, and the history clearly excludes acute viral pneumonitis or interstitial pulmonary edema. His symptoms suggest an asthma-like illness, but clinically he does not fit the description of a true asthmatic. The long history of wheezing and dyspnea, the absence of hemoptysis, and the normal laboratory data eliminate a type II immune response, leaving us with either a type III immune response, a lymphoproliferative disorder, or one of the chronic interstitial pneumonias as a possible diagnosis. In considering a type III immune response, it is usually easier to first eliminate the autoimmune diseases by history and physical examination. If the patient has no known collagen vascular disorder, a careful examination of his history must be made for a possible antigen. Elimination of the antigen from the patient's environment and proper treatment may save him from a progressive destructive pulmonary disease. The list of possible antigens is quite long, and new ones are constantly being added. In this case, the patient admitted that he had worked as a pigeon handler for many years and that the onset of the syptomatology coincided with that of his occupation. (A pigeon serum skin test carried out at a later date was positive.)

The patient was then lost to follow-up and was not seen until 10 years later, at which time he obviously had severe parenchymal interstitial fibrosis as well as cyst formation (Fig. E–7b). Figure E–7c was made approximately a year before the patient's demise. At autopsy, the pulmonary parenchyma was found to be widely and irregularly affected by a fibrosing and destructive process. The cause of death was pneumonia superimposed upon a fibrocystic disease of the lungs compatible with the clinical diagnosis of pigeon breeder's disease.

CASE E–8

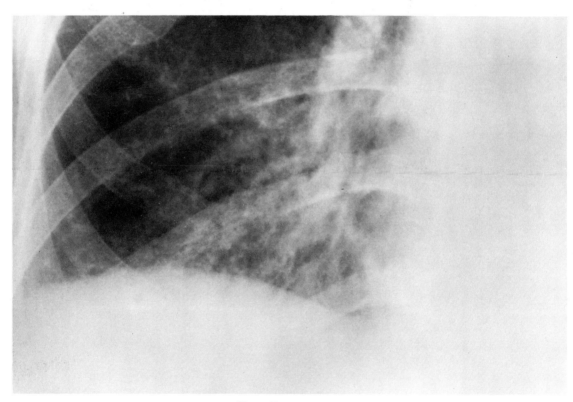

Figure E–8   Close-up

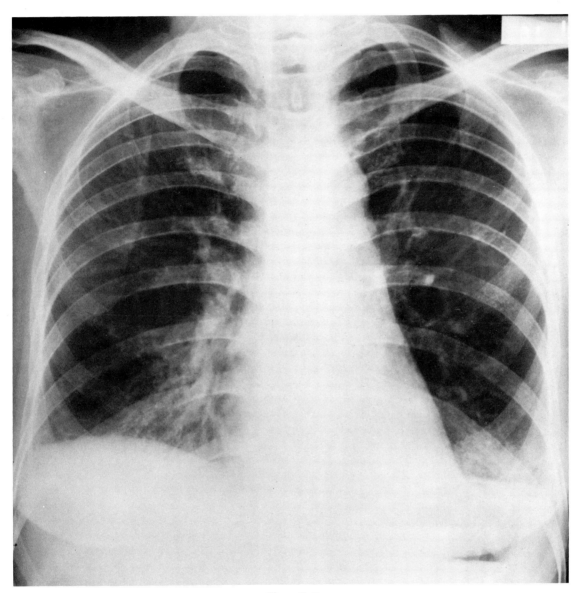

Figure E–8

Case E–8. This patient was a 40 year old Asian female who had a known chronic disease. You should be able to make this diagnosis.

DISCUSSION, CASE E–8

This is another case of progressive systemic sclerosis. The basilar fibrotic pattern seen in the radiograph of this middle-aged female is typical of this disease, and a patient with these changes almost certainly will have gastro-intestinal symptomatology and perhaps skin changes as well.

It is difficult to rule out superimposed pneumonitis in this type of patient, and the radiograph must be correlated with the clinical data. In the absence of new respiratory symptomatology or any other sign of infection, the changes noted in this patient are rather typical of progressive systemic sclerosis.

Occasionally, polymyositis or dermatomyositis may present a very simi-lar radiographic picture, with pulmonary fibrosis most marked in the lower lobes.

CASE E–9 _____

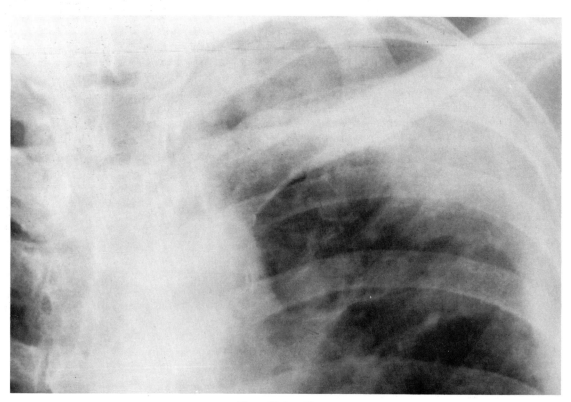

Figure E–9a Close-up

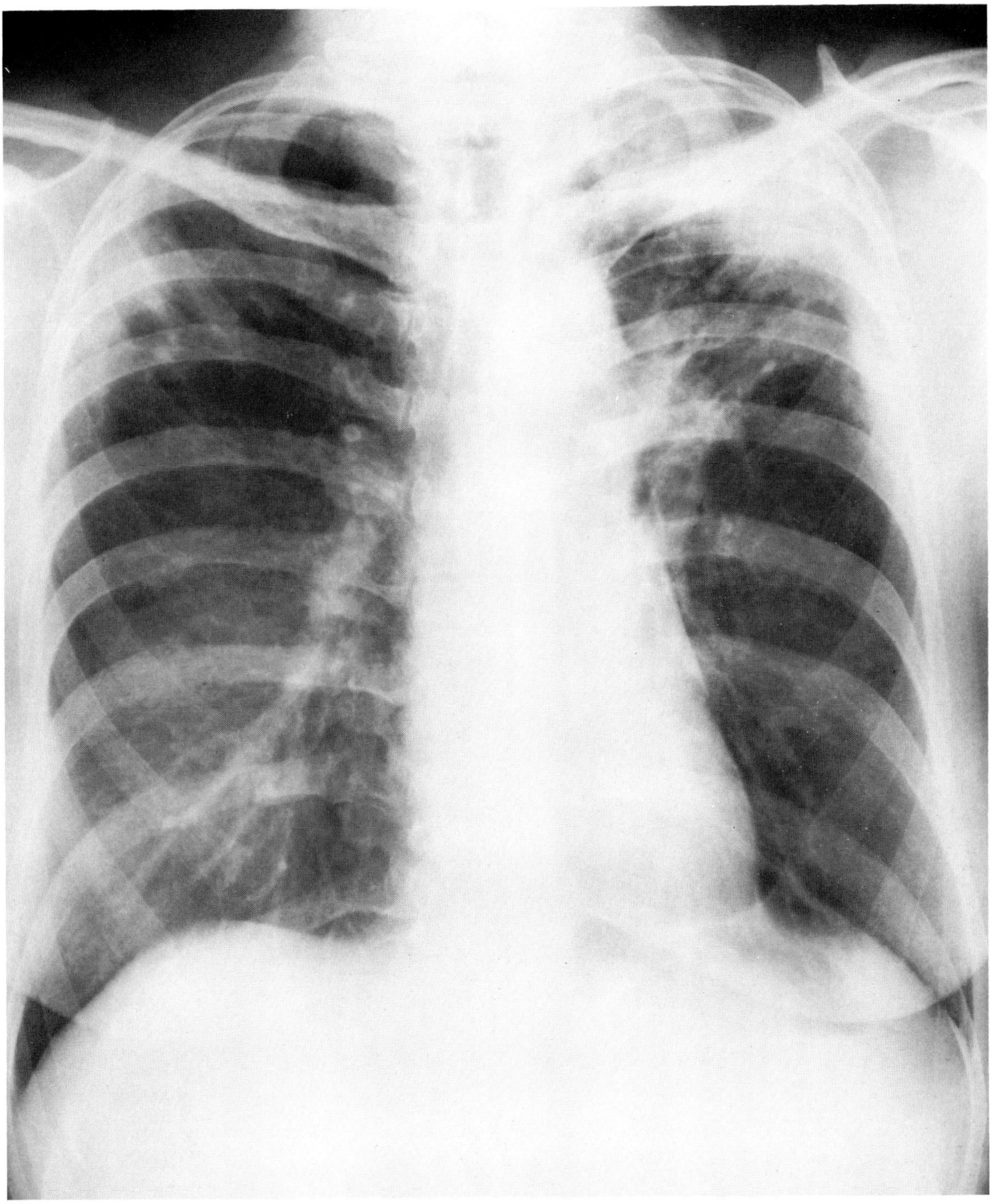

Figure E-9a

Case E-9a.   This patient was a 47 year old white female who presented with a nonproductive cough, a low-grade fever, moderate dyspnea, and chest discomfort. Her previous history was significant only in that she suffered from known multiple allergies. A skin test and multiple sputum smears were all negative for tuberculosis. What is your differential diagnosis? What additional laboratory information would you request?

Additional radiographs of this patient are demonstrated on the next two pages, but try to make the diagnosis before looking at them.

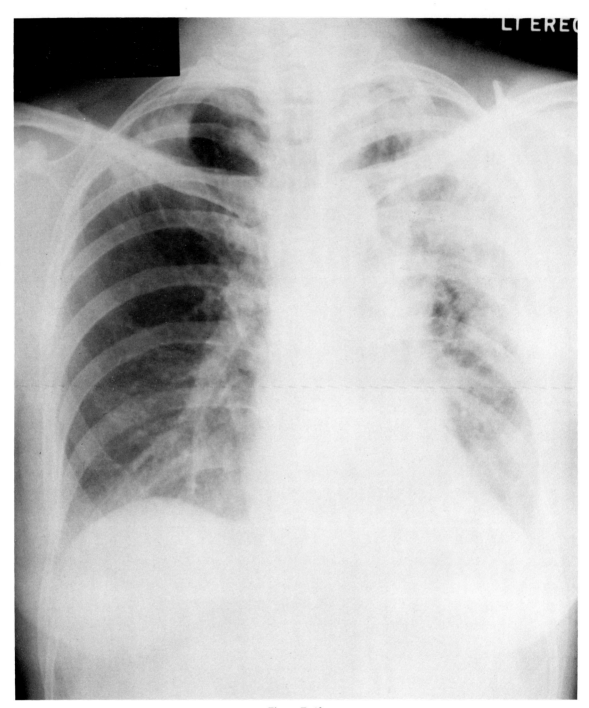

Figure E–9b

   Case E–9b. This radiograph of the same patient shown in Figure E–9a
was made approximately 3 weeks later.

Figure E–9c

Case E–9c. This radiograph was made of the same patient seen in Figures E–9a and E–9b after appropriate therapy.

DISCUSSION, CASE E–9

There are probably many of you who think that in this case tuberculosis cannot be excluded radiographically, and I agree. However, the negative skin test and sputum smears and the nonproductive cough make tuberculosis a quite unlikely diagnosis. If you would like to know whether the patient had blood eosinophilia, you're on the right track, as she had persistent and significant eosinophilia. The correct diagnosis is chronic eosinophilic pneumonia, which was cleared promptly by steroid therapy. This entity has been called pulmonary infiltrates with eosinophilia (PIE). It is a type III antigen-antibody reaction, and in cases of this disorder there is undoubtedly an inhaled antigen to which the patient reacts. One might think that a careful examination of the history would provide a clue that would identify the antigen, but some cases with a type III antigen-antibody reaction defy a definite diagnosis. Fortunately, the condition is usually cleared rapidly and completely by steroid therapy, but recurrences have been noted.

The often typical radiographic picture shows a peripheral interstitial and at times alveolar filling process, and it is most often bilateral, as in Figure E–9a. The intensity of the inflammatory reaction in the left lung is indicated by the upward retraction of the hilum, and this change also makes one think of tuberculosis. Some observers have found the peripheral nature of the disease so striking that it has been called the "negative" of pulmonary edema.

CASE E–10

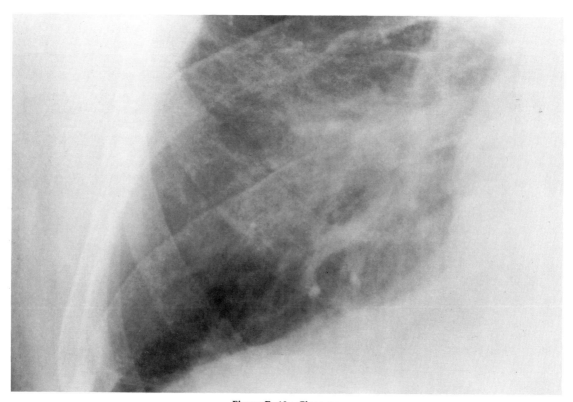

Figure E–10 Close-up

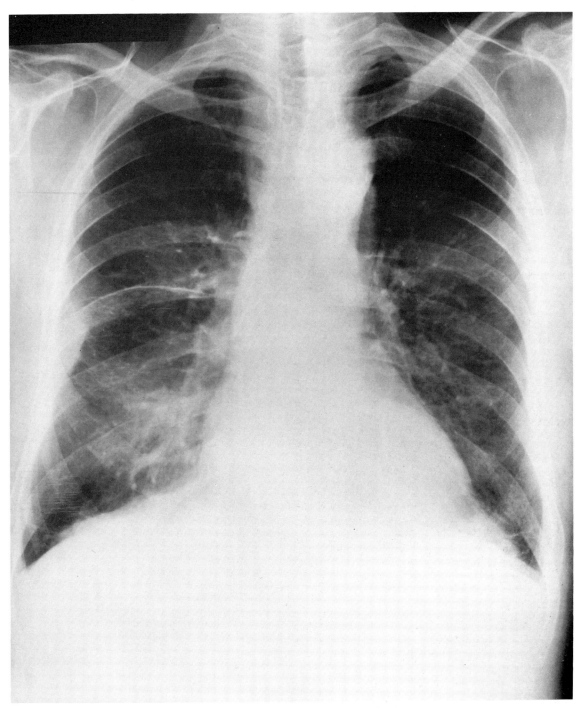

Figure E–10

Case E–10. This patient was a 70 year old white male who presented for a routine examination and complained only of minor dyspnea on exertion. What is your diagnosis?

DISCUSSION, CASE E–10

The radiographic changes seen in this case are virtually pathognomonic, and the diagnosis is asbestosis. Over 90 per cent of patients who have any evidence of thoracic asbestosis will have pleural plaques. A parenchymal fibrotic reaction without pleural thickening is quite unusual. In asbestosis both the pleural disease and the parenchymal interstitial changes are almost always confined to the lower half of the chest. Close observation of the radiograph presented in Figure E–10 also reveals a calcified pleural plaque in the left hemidiaphragm. Pathologists have found most of these calcifications in the diaphragmatic muscle itself. Less frequently, plaques along the lateral thoracic pleura calcify as well. The longer the time that has elapsed since the exposure to asbestos fibers, the more likely it is that calcification will be present. The only other industrial disease to be included in the differential diagnosis is talcosis, and some observers believe that it is actually the asbestos-like chemical composition of some talc that is the cause of this similar pulmonary disease. Very rarely, widespread healed tuberculosis must be considered in the differential diagnosis, but the distribution of the parenchymal as well as the pleural changes is usually quite different in this condition.

At times, the history of exposure to asbestos is difficult to obtain, and many older patients have to be questioned about their occupations during the Second World War, as the pulmonary changes caused by asbestos can be acquired in a relatively short period of time.

The incidence of neoplasm in patients with asbestosis is exceedingly high in those who smoke, and the neoplasm is most commonly a bronchogenic carcinoma. In such patients, the incidence of mesothelioma, peritoneal as well as pleural, is also markedly increased over that in the general population.

CASE E–11

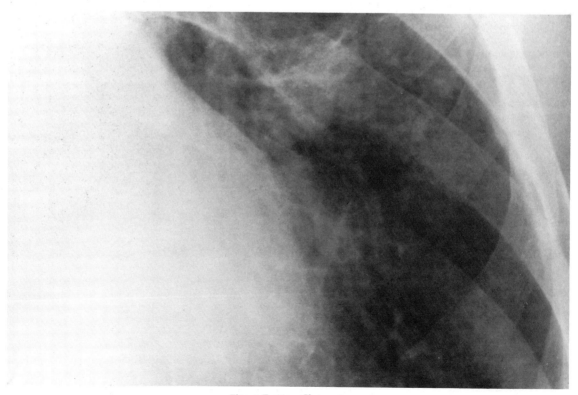

Figure E–11a   Close-up

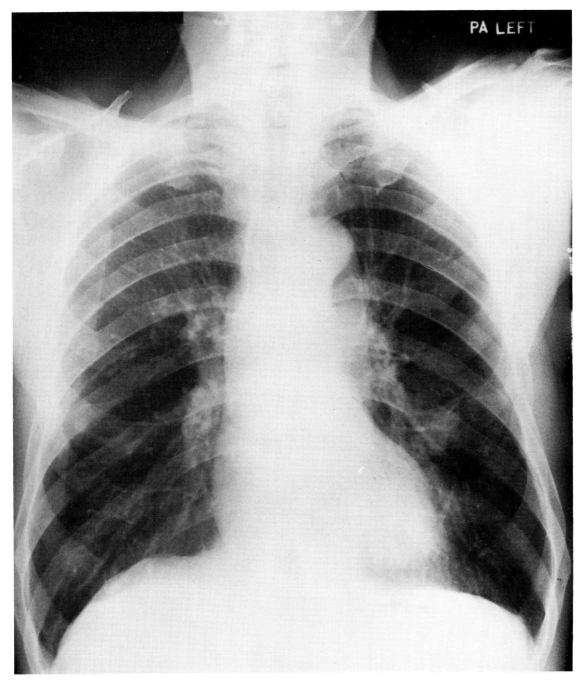

Figure E–11a

Case E–11a. This patient was a 72 year old white male who presented for a routine chest examination. Try to make the diagnosis before turning the page. A radiograph made 3 years later is demonstrated on the next page.

CASE E–11 *CONTINUED*

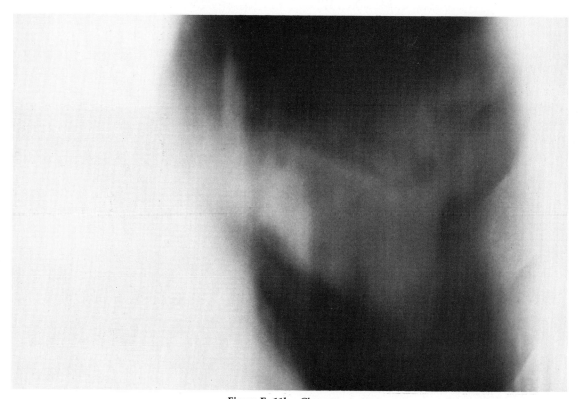

Figure E–11b   Close-up

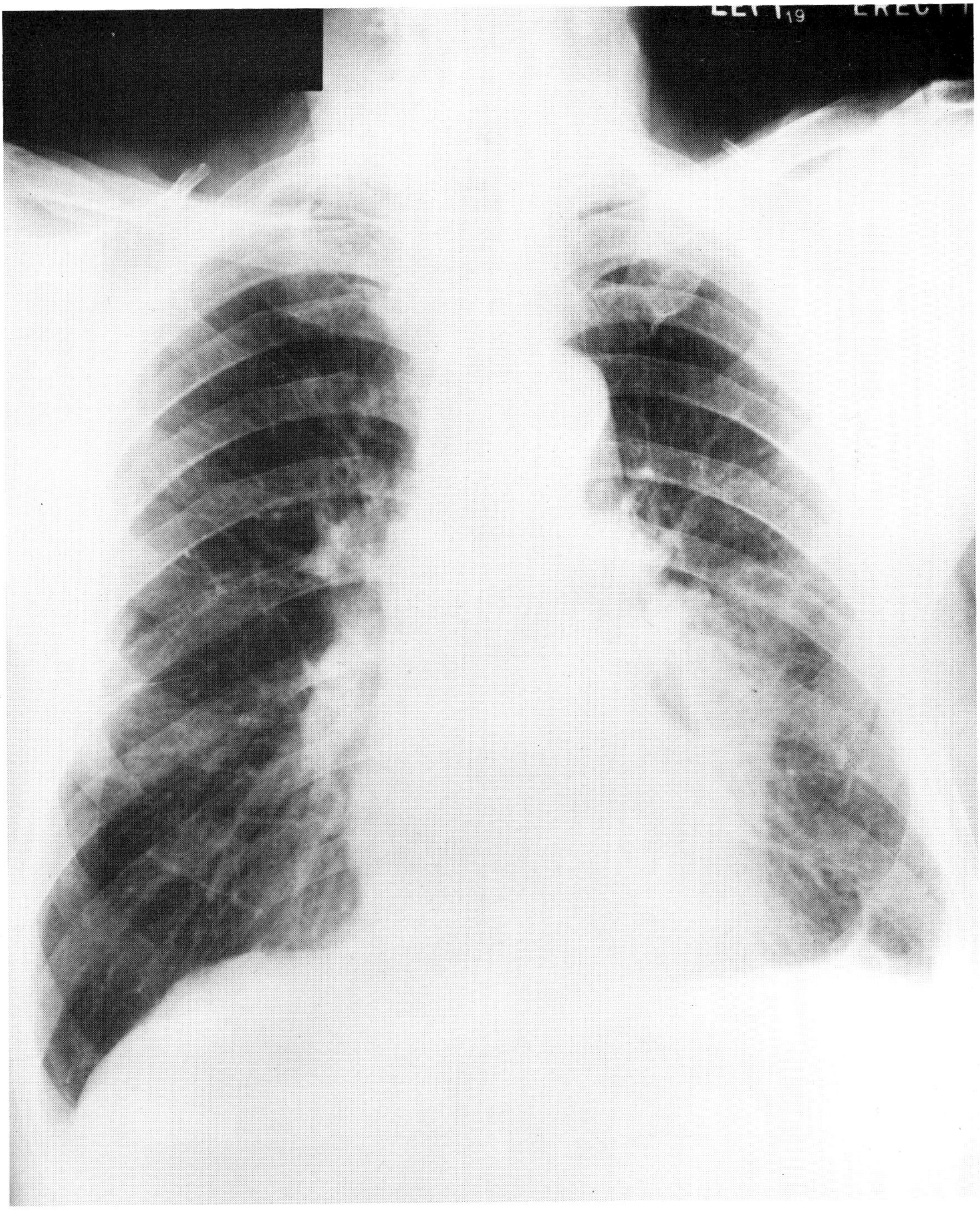

Figure E-11b

Case E-11b. This radiograph of the same patient shown in Figure E-11a was made 3 years later. The close-up (Fig. E-11b) is a tomogram made of the left mid-chest.

DISCUSSION, CASE E–11

If you made the diagnosis of asbestosis, you are correct but only partially so. The small lesion seen in Figure E–11a in the left infrahilar area is a bronchogenic carcinoma not appreciated at the time the radiograph was made. The mass on the left side is quite obvious in the radiograph made 3 years later, but it is also obviously slow-growing. Tomograms made at the time of original radiograph 3 years earlier would almost certainly have demonstrated the mass, and needless to say, a diagnosis made at that time would have made a significant difference to the patient. The lesson in this case is that one must develop a very high index of suspicion with patients who have radiographic manifestations of asbestosis, particularly if the patient smokes or has in the past.

CASE E–12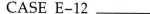

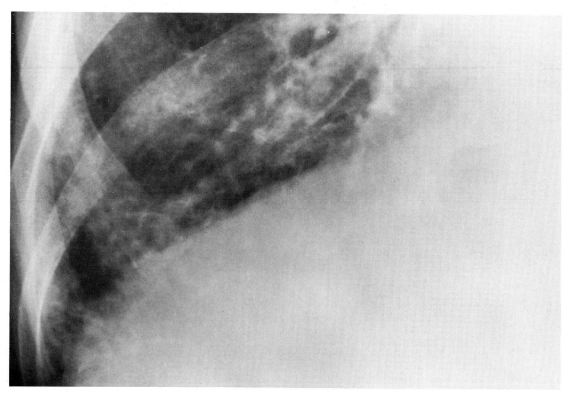

Figure E–12   Close-up

Figure E–12

Case E–12. This patient was a 65 year old white male who presented with increasingly severe dyspnea on exertion and a known chronic disease.

DISCUSSION, CASE E–12

The diagnosis is unfortunately obvious. The patient has a large left effusion that is irregular in its upper portion, because of either loculation or pleural-based masses. The close-up of the right lower lobe demonstrates the pleural thickening and parenchymal fibrosis compatible with a diagnosis of asbestosis. The combination of the findings on each side of the chest leads to the final diagnosis of malignant mesothelioma. Although the most common neoplasm that develops in asbestos workers is bronchogenic carcinoma, the increase in the incidence of mesothelioma in these workers in relation to that in the general population is much greater than the increase in the incidence of bronchogenic carcinoma. Some patients will develop mesotheliomas of the peritoneum rather than of the pleura.

In a significant percentage of the general population, studies done at autopsy have found ferruginous bodies containing fibers. However, careful investigation has proven that many of the fibers within the iron-containing gelatinous capsules are not asbestos fibers, and there is no firm evidence at this time that asbestos fibers are harmful to the general population.

CASE E–13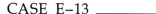

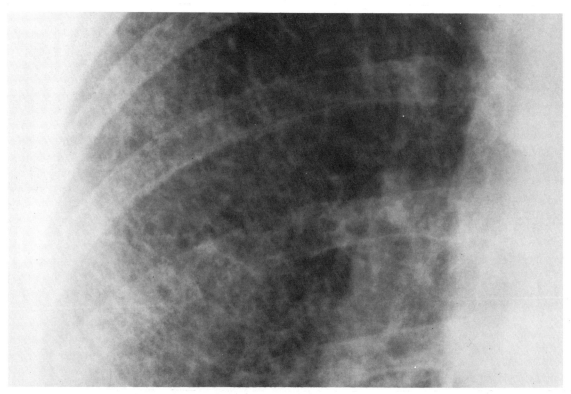

Figure E–13 Close-up

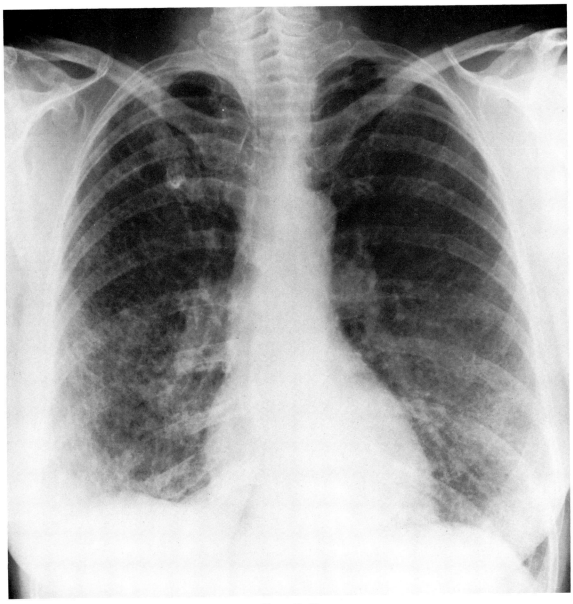

Figure E-13

Case E-13. This patient was a 58 year old white female who presented with 1 year of increasing dyspnea, a moderate cough, and questionable cyanosis. Laboratory data revealed moderate anemia and an abnormal serum protein electrophoretogram. (This case is included courtesy of Jean-Paul Bierny, M.D., Tucson, Arizona.)

Case E-13 will be discussed along with Case E-14, which is similar in etiology. What diagnosis would you consider in these two cases?

CASE E–14

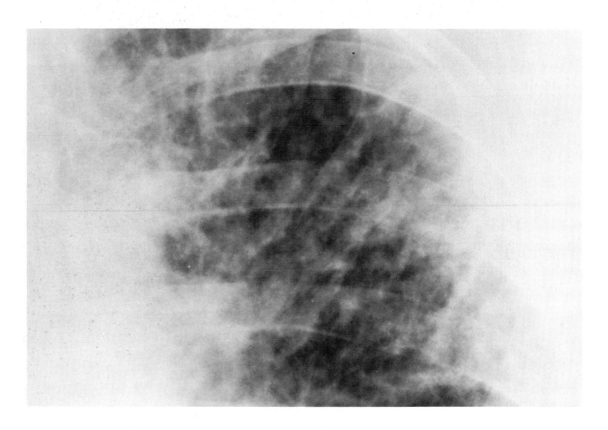

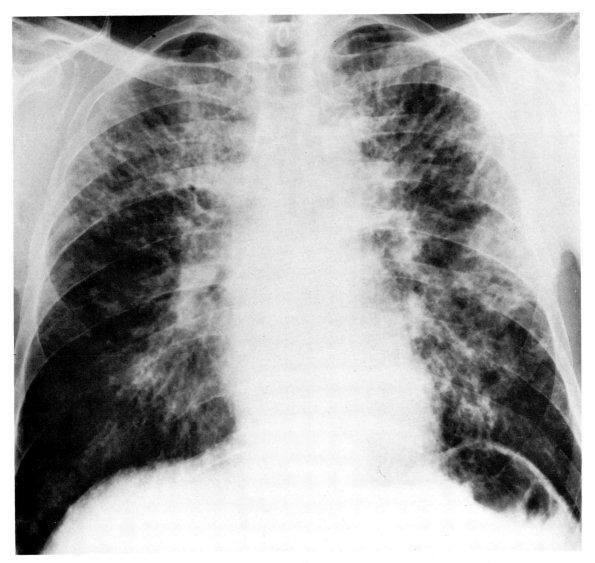

Figure E-14

Case E-14.   This patient was a 61 year old white male who presented after several months of fatigue, weight loss, dyspnea, and peripheral edema. He was treated initially at another institution with digitalis and diuretics, with a good response. Not long thereafter, however, his symptomatology became progressively more severe. Serum electrophoresis of this patient's blood was also abnormal. The correct diagnosis in this case is similar but not identical to that in Case E-13.

DISCUSSION, CASES E–13 and E–14

The specific diagnosis for the patient shown in Figure E–13 is Waldenström's macroglobulinemia. Lung biopsy revealed an interstitial infiltration with plasmacytoid cells and very minimal fibrosis. The diagnosis in Case E–14 is primary systemic amyloidosis with a monoclonal gammopathy. Analysis of this patient's urinary proteins by immunoelectrophoresis revealed a monoclonal lambda light chain peak. At autopsy the patient was found to have diffuse primary amyloidosis of all organs examined and to have actually died of heart failure secondary to amyloid myocardiopathy.

The two diseases just mentioned are related to each other and to multiple myeloma because all three involve an abnormality of the B lymphocyte. Lung biopsies performed on patients with Waldenström's macroglobulinemia typically reveal infiltration with plasmacytoid lymphocytes, with minimal fibrosis, if any, and without amyloidosis. Some authors believe primary amyloidosis should be included in the group of plasma cell dyscrasias because the B lymphocyte is again responsible for producing the abnormal light chain fragments of immunoglobulin characteristic of the disease.

CASE E–15

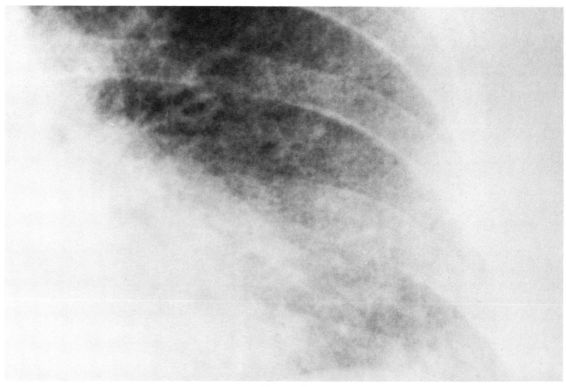

Figure E–15 Close-up

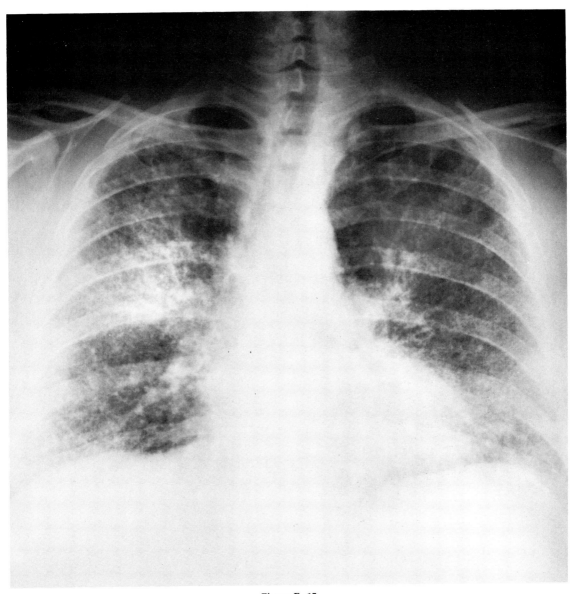

Figure E–15

Case E–15. This patient was a 54 year old white male who presented with moderate but increasing dyspnea on exertion. He had no significant past history, and all laboratory data were within normal limits. Despite careful questioning, no exposure to any known antigen could be discovered. The next patient, Case E–16, had the same disease. Both cases will be discussed on page 230. What is your differential diagnosis in these two cases?

CASE E–16

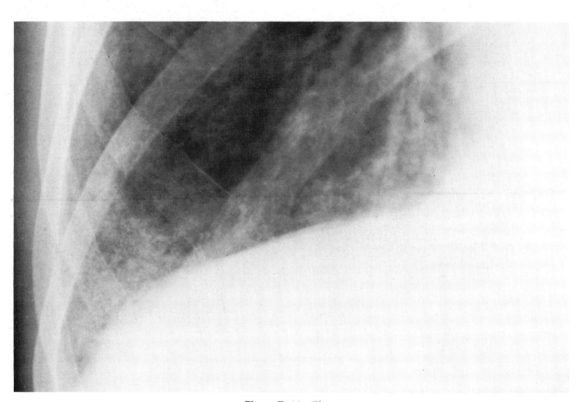

Figure E–16   Close-up

Figure E–16

Case E–16. This patient was a 42 year old white male who presented with only moderate dyspnea. There were no significant historical facts or laboratory data. (The radiograph suggests the possibility of a cavity in the left lower lobe, but none was found.)

DISCUSSION, CASES E–15 and E–16

Both patients have interstitial disease, possibly fibrotic. In the first patient the disease is diffuse, and in the second it is limited to the lung bases. Biopsy in each case revealed desquamative interstitial pneumonia. Originally, it was thought that this disease was confined to the lung bases. In this observer's experience, however, the diffuse pattern seen in Figure E–15 is more common. To establish the diagnosis, it is almost always necessary to perform a lung biopsy, in which large desquamated alveolar cells are typically found.

CASE E–17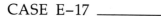

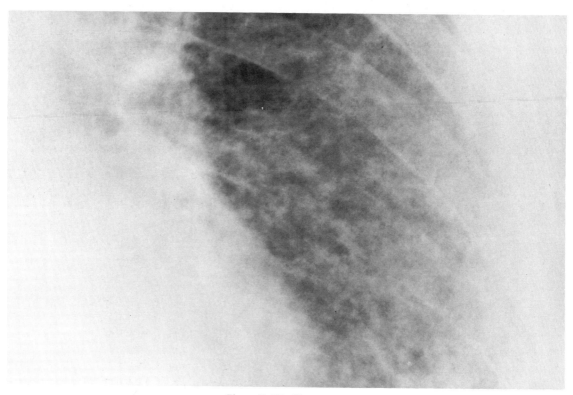

Figure E–17   Close-up

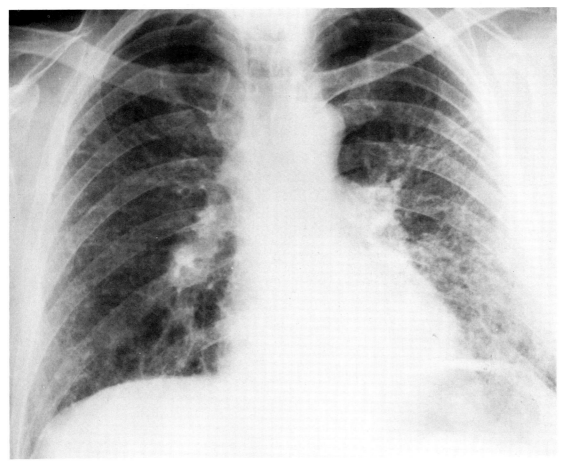

Figure E–17

Case E–17. This patient was a 62 year old white male who presented with dyspnea that had increased during the several weeks prior to admission. The patient had a history of coronary atherosclerotic disease, but despite digitalis and diuretic therapy, his shortness of breath continued to increase in severity. Blood gas analysis revealed a moderately low oxygen saturation. There were no other significant historical, physical, or laboratory data. How would you diagnose this case before lung biopsy? (This case is included courtesy of Jean-Paul Bierny, M.D., Tucson, Arizona.)

DISCUSSION, CASE E–17

In this case the lung biopsy alone did not establish the diagnosis, but as expected, it revealed diffuse pulmonary interstitial fibrosis. The progressive clinical symptomatology, the radiographic appearance, and the lung biopsy lead to the clinical diagnosis of the Hamman-Rich syndrome. This case also fits the diagnosis of usual interstitial pneumonia (UIP) of the Liebow classification of which the Hamman-Rich syndrome is the clinically progressive variety.

CASE E–18 _____

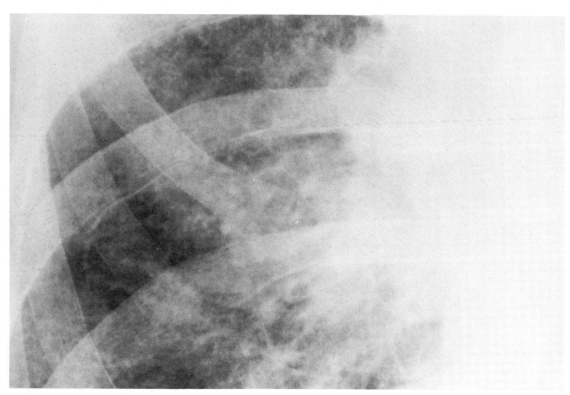

Figure E–18   Close-up

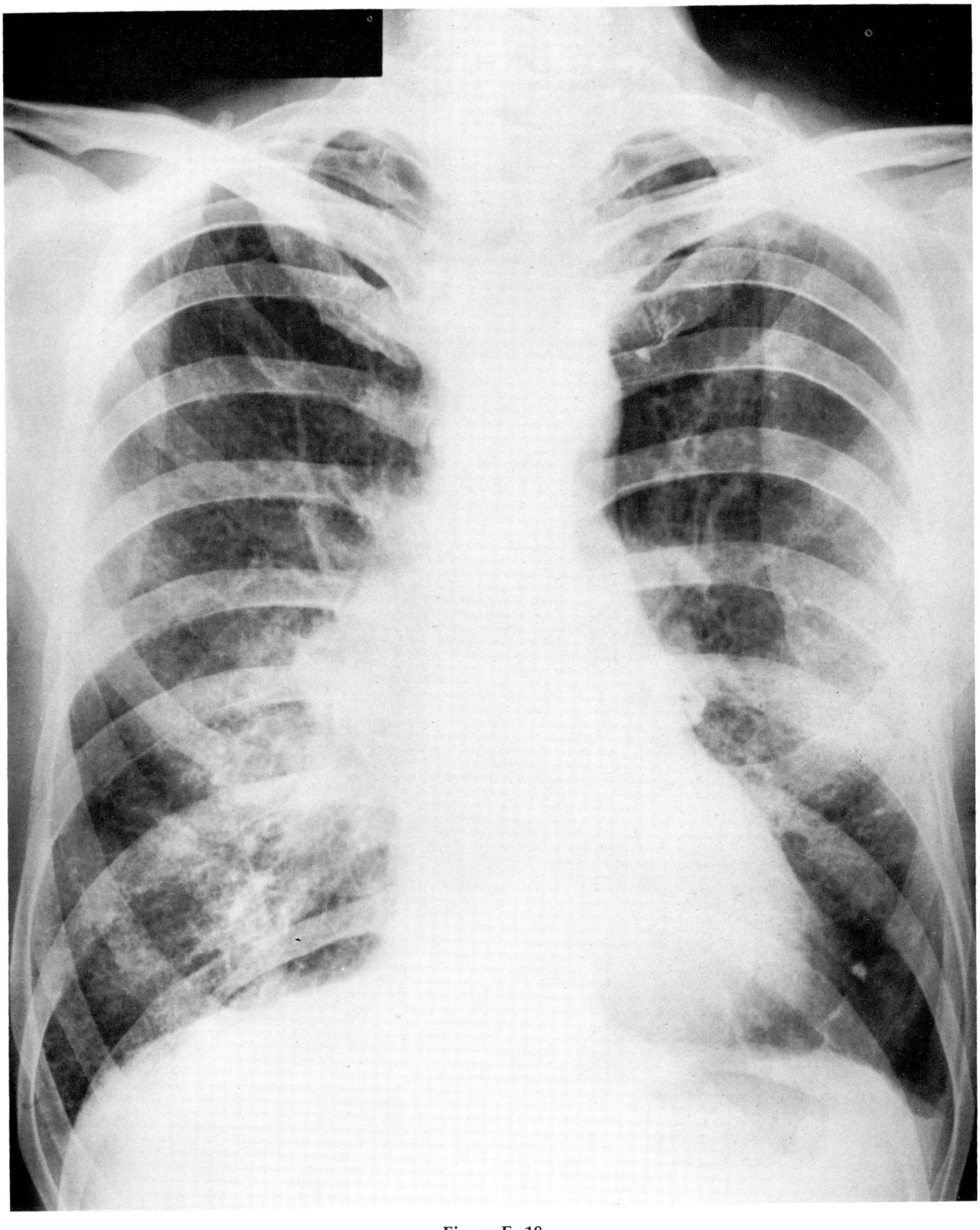

Figure E-18

Case E-18. This patient was a 54 year old white male who presented with moderate dyspnea on exertion, a nonproductive cough, and one episode of hemoptysis. Physical examination and laboratory data were noncontributory. Use this case as a final unknown, and see if you can formulate the precise diagnosis.

DISCUSSION, CASE E–18

Did you note the pleural thickening in each costophrenic angle and the interstitial disease in the lower half of the thorax? If you want to know whether the patient has an industrial history or whether he has been exposed to asbestos dust, you are correct in suspecting that he has asbestosis. The calcifications on the left side of the chest are not related to this disease and are not significant, but the large right hilum contains a bronchogenic carcinoma and is almost certainly secondary to this patient's known asbestosis.

REFERENCES

1. Bruwer, A., Kennedy, R. L. J., and, Edwards, J.: Recurrent pulmonary hemorrhage with hemosiderosis: so-called idiopathic pulmonary hemosiderosis. Am. J. Roentgenol., 76:98–107, 1956.
2. Carrington, C. B., Gaensler, E. A., Coutu, R. E., et al.: Natural history and treated course of usual and desquamative interstitial pneumonia. N. Engl. J. Med., 298(15):801–809, 1978.
3. Frazier, A. R., and Miller, R.D.: Interstitial pneumonitis in association with polymyositis and dermatomyositis. Chest, 65:403–407, 1974.
4. Feigin, D. S., Siegelman, S. S., Theros, E. G., et al.: Nonmalignant lymphoid disorders of the chest. Am. J. Roentgenol., 129:221–228, 1977.
5. Feldman, F., Ellis, K., and Green, W.: The fat embolism syndrome. Radiology, 114:535–542, 1975.
6. Heitzman, E. R., Markarian, B., and DeLise, C. T.: Lymphoproliferative disorders of the tho-
7. Herman, P., Balikian, J., Seltzer, S., and Ehrie, M.: The Pulmonary-Renal Syndrome. Am. J. Roentgenol., 130:1141–1148, 1978.
8. Liebow, A. A., Steer, A., and Billingsley, J.: Desquamative interstitial pneumonia. Am. J. Med., 39:369–404, 1965.
9. Malik, S. K., Pardee, N., and Martin, C.: Involvement of the lungs in tuberous sclerosis. Chest, 58:538–539, 1970.
10. McCombs, R.: Diseases due to immunologic reactions in the lungs. 1. N. Engl. J. Med., 286(22):1186–1194, 1972.
11. McCombs, R.: Diseases due to immunologic reactions in the lungs. 2. N. Engl. J. Med., 186(23):1245–1252, 1972.
12. Mindell, H.: Roentgen findings in farmer's lung. Radiology, 97:341–346, 1970.
13. Nam, K., and Gracey, D.: Pulmonary talcosis from cosmetic talcum powder. JAMA, 221:492–493, 1972.
14. Petty, T., and Wilkins, M.: Five manifestations of rheumatoid lung. Dis. Chest, 49:1–66, 1975.
15. Popper, M., Bogdonoff, M. L., and Hughes, R. L.: Interstitial rheumatoid lung disease. Chest, 62:243–250, 1972.
16. Roberts, S. R.: Immunology and the lung: an overview. Semin. Roentgenol., 10(1):7–19, 1975.
17. Sargent, E. N., Jacobson, G., and Gordonson, J. S.: Pleural plaques: a signpost of asbestos dust inhalation. Semin. Roentgenol., 12:287–297, 1977.
18. Schwartz, E. E., and Holsclaw, D. S.: Pulmonary involvement in adults with cystic fibrosis. Am. J. Roentgenol., 122:708–718, 1974.
19. Schwartz, E. E., Teplick, J. G., Onesti, G., et al.: Pulmonary hemorrhage in renal disease: Goodpasture's syndrome and other causes. Radiology, 122:39–46, 1977.
20. Selikoff, I. J., and Churg, J.: Biological effects of asbestos. Ann. N.Y. Acad. Sci., 132:1–766, 1965.
21. Selikoff, I. J., Hammond, E. C., and Churg, J.: Asbestos exposure, smoking and neoplasia. JAMA, 204:104–110, 1968.
22. Siegelman, S. S.: Plasma cell dyscrasias. In Jacobson, H. G., and Murray, J. F. (eds.): The Radiology of Skeletal Disorders: Exercises in Diagnosis, 2nd ed. New York, Longman, Inc., 1977.
23. Unger, J., Fink, J., and Unger, G.: Pigeon breeder's disease. Radiology, 90:683–687, 1968.
24. Unger, G. F., Scanlon, G. T., Fink, J. N., et al.: A radiologic approach to hypersensitivity pneumonias. Radiol. Clin. North Am., 11(2):339–356, 1973.
25. Wolson, A. H., and Rohwedder, J. J.: Upper lobe fibrosis in ankylosing spondylitis. Am. J. Roentgenol., 124:466–471, 1975.

Index